50 Things That Cause Heart Attack

Padma Sundareson

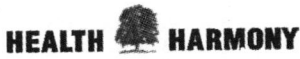

An imprint of
B. Jain Publishers (P) Ltd.
USA — Europe — India

Disclaimer

Any information given in this book is not intended to be taken as a replacement for medical advice. Any person with a condition requiring medical attention should consult a qualified practitioner or therapist.

50 THINGS THAT CAUSE HEART ATTACK

First Edition: 2012
1st Impression: 2012

All rights reserved. No part of this book may be reproduced, stored in a retrieval system or transmitted, in any form or by any means, mechanical, photocopying, recording or otherwise, without any prior written permission of the publisher.

© with author

Published by Kuldeep Jain for

HEALTH HARMONY

An imprint of
B. JAIN PUBLISHERS (P) LTD.
1921/10, Chuna Mandi, Paharganj, New Delhi 110 055 (INDIA)
Tel.: +91-11-4567 1000 • *Fax:* +91-11-4567 1010
Email: info@bjain.com • *Website:* **www.bjain.com**

Printed in India by
J.J. Offset Printers

ISBN: 978-81-319-1143-3

Preface

*'A joyful heart is the inevitable result of
a heart burning with Love.'*

– Mother Teresa

All human emotions are associated to the heart. A heart racing with excitement simply proves this fact. The Heart is an integral part of our body. No one can live without a heart.

We all know that the heart is a very strong pump that sends blood to the entire body. The blood vessels that supply the heart are called Coronary Arteries. When this pumping system gets clogged up, there is a lack of blood supply to the heart. The urgency of repair depends on the severity of the blockage. A total blockage of the coronary artery stops complete blood flow to the heart muscles. This causes a heart attack.

Heart disease is the number one cause of death around the world. According to an article in the *Indian Heart Journal*, half a million people have heart attacks each year in the United States and India has 60 per cent. Which shows that we have 60 per cent of the world's heart disease.

FEAR is the prime emotion associated with heart attacks. Anyone who had a 'Myocardial infarction or heart attack' is petrified and naturally wants to know what has caused this terrible ordeal in his life. Knowing the cause brings a certain amount of reassurance and a hope to fight back.

By writing this book, I trust that people will learn something new about the causes of heart attack. Knowledge and education makes prevention of this deadly disease possible.

An heart attack can be life altering, but with necessary lifestyle changes and medications we can bring it back on track. Motivate yourself. Anyone who has survived an attack should realise that it is by no means the end of life. It is one big opportunity to realise what went wrong and take full control of your life.

Some of you are perhaps reading this book, because you have been diagnosed with coronary artery disease and would like to prevent a heart attack. There are several ongoing researches on heart attacks today. Thanks to the advances, scientists are able to pinpoint even the most remote causes. Medical professionals are adept in treating heart attacks quickly. But remember – Prevention is the Key.

Every small change matters. Concentrate on reversing the reversible risk factors. Smoking is a definite – No. The toxins in cigarettes directly affect arteries and heart. Eat sensibly. Keep your blood pressure normal. Avoid or minimize foods that are high in fat and sugar. Maintain a healthy weight and exercise at least 30 minutes a day.

There is no bigger gift in life than life itself. So, make the most of it.

Padma Sundareson

Acknowledgements

I am indebted to the Lord Almighty for bestowing his blessings and grace to guide me all through the way.

I owe an enormous debt of gratitude to my family's constant support that made it possible for this book to happen. A special thanks to my brother Arun and my cousin Sukanya for reading this manuscript with a critical eye.

I am grateful to Ms Inara Hasanali for introducing me to the B Jain Publishing, offering valuable suggestions and guiding me.

I would like to thank Dr Geeta Rani Arora for giving me the splendid opportunity to write this book. I thank all the team members of B Jain Publishing, who helped to get this book published.

I wish to thank all my near and dear ones for their well wishes.

Padma Sundareson

Publisher's Note

'Heart attack…is the leading killer of mankind today.'

It is very important to be aware and recognise the symptoms of a heart attack, immediately. There are countless physical signs which are mild and people tend to ignore. Typically, this painful experience is hard to disregard.

This book has been designed to be a perfect guide for all heart problems. It has some very interesting points for the readers to make them self comprised about their all round awareness regarding – the heart.

Why not develop the security you crave from others by reading and finding it out – yourself? Why not provide the nurturing you long for?

Read the book and develop your own wisdom yourself – for you life ahead.

Kuldeep Jain
C.E.O., B. Jain Publishers (P) Ltd.

Contents

Preface — *iii*
Acknowledgements — *vi*
Publisher's Note — *vii*

1. Introduction — 1
2. Know Your Heart — 5
3. What Happens during a Heart Attack — 11
4. 50 Causes of a Heart Attack — 19
5. Tests to Diagnose Coronary Artery Disease — 129
6. Treatment Options — 145
7. Complications of a Heart Attack — 161
8. Prevention — 171
9. Cardio Pulmonary Resuscitation (CPR) — 179
   Glossary — 184
   References — 189

Chapter 1

Introduction

> *It was a monday morning, I was getting ready to work... Everything seemed usual except some chest tightness and uneasiness in my stomach. I was just out of the door when I felt pressure, like an elephant sitting on my chest knocking the wind out of me... I was having a heart attack...*

Heart attacks are not uncommon. It is considered the leading killer of mankind, claiming 17.1 million lives each year. A heart attack is sometimes the first time a man ever finds out that he had ongoing heart disease. A blockage only few millimetres in diameter could pose enormous threat to his life. More than one in three adults is being diagnosed with a heart disease.

It is estimated that in USA, about 1.5 million people suffer a heart attack every year. Over 30 per cent of these people die. In 2010, India is supposed to bear 60 per cent of the world's heart disease.

We find that books and media are filled with numbers and per centages. It may sometimes create a sense of validity or just generate confusion. These statistics are not given to scare anyone but warns us to take charge of our heart health. As an individual do not let numbers rule your worries. Your risk factors are exclusive to you and needs to be discussed with your doctor. Regular annual checkups are a good way to diagnose early and keep the worst at bay.

Heart attack can be devastating to your life and your families. The purpose of this book is to provide knowledge and awareness. You can make a difference to your heart health.

About 70 per cent people are still out there after a heart attack struggling to pull their lives back together. With advancing gains in modern medicine there is a better hope for recovery. Life after a heart attack can be a battle, but it should not be a compromise. Life can pass you by unless you take charge. Prevention is the greatest chance we have to overcome this impending doom.

The heart muscles die if left without any blood for a very long time. Early intervention can limit or avoid permanent injury to the heart muscles and even prevent complications. Hence, it is crucial to recognise the signs of a heart attack and act immediately. Delay in such cases can be deadly.

It is essential to get to an emergency care at the earliest. Doctors can clear the block in the artery and restore blood supply to the injured heart muscles. Treatments do not stop once you leave the hospital. It is not only necessary to take medications without fail, but it is vital to make some necessary changes in lifestyle.

'Lifestyle Modification' is now a commonly used and heard phrase. It is difficult to change our comfortable lifestyles overnight. Is it worth pursuing smoking, eating fat rich foods or being inactive if it can double or even triple your chances of heart attacks? Think about it. Why suffer that pain? Would anyone like to take several pills everyday to keep their heart pumping effectively, when the need could have been avoided? Leading a healthy life starts early, as early as childhood.

Now most adults already have some amount of blockage in their coronary arteries. The size may be very small to cause any shortage of blood supply to the heart. Nevertheless, good lifestyle can prevent further damage. People with existing heart conditions should continue their regular visits to the doctor, eat their pills regularly, be active and do all what they can to avoid a heart attack.

Taking care of your heart and leading a healthy life is not a day's work but a life long commitment.

Chapter 2
Know Your Heart

We all know that heart is one of the major organs of the human body. The heart is located in the middle of the chest, slightly to the left below the sternum. Its average size is about the size of a man's fist or slightly larger. The heart is the first organ to be formed and starts beating at about 22 days after conception. On an average a normal heart beats about 72 times per minute, pumping blood to the entire body.

The heart has three layers:

- Epicardium – outermost layer of the heart
- Myocardium – middle layer of the heart. It is made up of powerful muscles which contracts and propels blood out
- Endocardium – innermost layer of the heart that lines the heart chambers

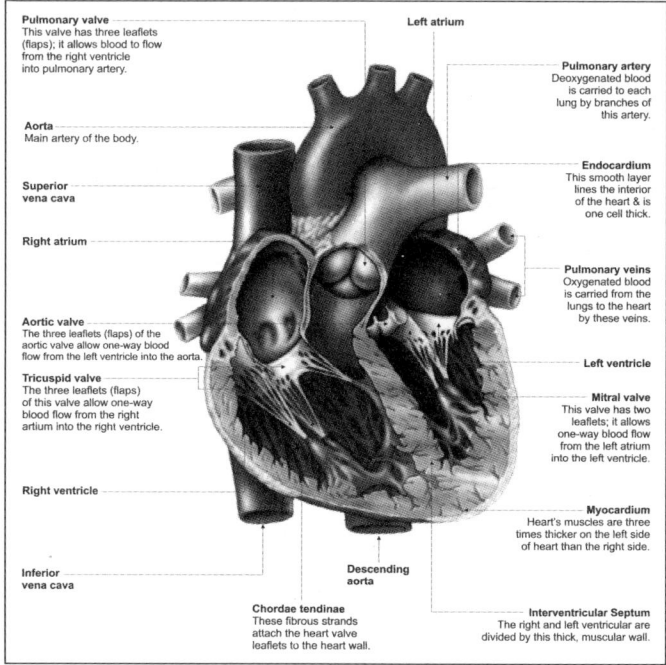

Fig. 2.1 View of the Heart

The heart has four chambers. The upper chambers are called atria and the lower chambers are called ventricles. The wall that divides the left and the right side of the heart is called the septum. There are four valves that regulate unidirectional flow of the blood and prevent any back flow. They are:

1. Mitral Valve – between the left atrium and left ventricle.
2. Tricuspid Valve – between the right atrium and right ventricle.
3. Pulmonary Valve – between the right ventricle and the main pulmonary artery.
4. Aortic Valve – between the left ventricle and the aorta.

The right side of the heart receives impure or deoxygenated blood from the body and pumps it to the lungs. Oxygen is infused into the blood in the lungs and is then sent to the left side of the heart. Aorta, the largest artery carries the oxygen rich blood from the left ventricle. It branches into several smaller arteries that supply oxygen rich blood to every single cell from head to toe.

Coronary Arteries

The first branch of aorta, rising right above the aortic valve is called the coronary artery.

'Coronary' is a word originating from Latin which means 'crown'. Like a crown these arteries can be seen on top of the heart. They branch, twine and supply oxygen and nutrients to the heart muscles or the myocardium

There are two main coronary arteries – the right and the left. The left coronary artery branches early into Left Anterior Descending artery and Left Circumflex Artery. Each branch supplies to a particular portion of the myocardium and the septum. The coronary supply varies from person to person.

Coronary Artery Disease

Having understood what the heart's basic structures and functions are, let us see what happens when a coronary artery is narrowed or blocked.

Coronary artery disease is the leading cause of death worldwide. The first stage of a coronary artery disease is called Atherosclerosis. Athero means artery and sclerosis means hardening of tissue.

Fatty materials and cell waste products often accumulate along the artery walls. This destructive process starts gradually and sometimes even as early as in our teenage years. Arteries become thick and rigid. Calcium deposits can occur. The coronary arteries narrow. Eventually, the blood flowing to the myocardium is decreased. This stage where the heart muscles are deprived of oxygen is termed as Myocardial Ischemia. People often have chest pain or angina, abnormal heart beats and syncope. The muscles are still not dead and this condition is often reversible.

Complete blockage of coronary artery causes a full stop of blood flowing to the myocardium. Continuous deprivation of oxygen will result in necrosis or cell death and is irreversible. This is called Myocardial Infarction or Heart Attack.

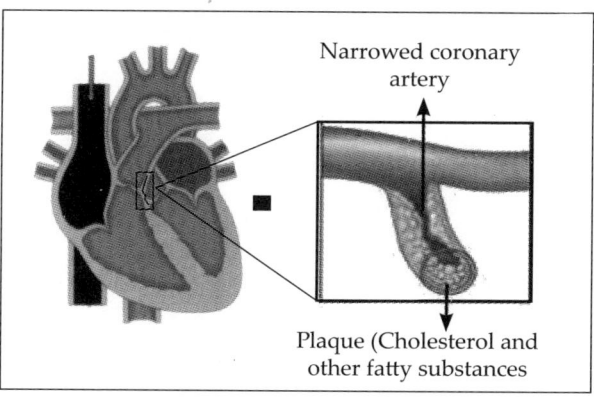

Fig. 2.2 Coronary Artery Disease

Chapter 3

What Happens during a Heart Attack

Atherosclerosis causes plaque to accumulate in the coronary arteries over a period of time. Earlier, it was thought that the main reason for heart attacks were these hard plaques blocking majority of the artery. Surprisingly, it is found that soft plaques in its early stages that do not narrow the artery lumen or does not interfere in blood supply may be unstable and are prone to rupture. A rupture causes blood clot formation resulting in an acute occlusion of the coronary arteries. Hence soft plaques are also called as 'Vulnerable Plaques'. In people with soft plaque build-up, the presence of coronary artery disease may not be detected until when presented as a heart attack.

Symptoms of a Heart Attack

It is important to be aware and recognise the symptoms of a heart attack immediately. There are countless physical signs which are mild and people tend to ignore. Typically this painful experience is hard to disregard.

The most common symptom of a heart attack is chest discomfort. The discomfort can be pain, pressure, tightness in the chest. The pain may be sharp or a crushing sensation in the left side that may travel to the neck, jaw, left arm and between the shoulder blades. The pain can be so powerful that it might not allow the person to breathe. At times it can just be a dull and persistent ache.

During a heart attack, the portion of the left ventricle that is affected does not efficiently pump out all the blood. Even, the area around the affected myocardium goes into a state of hibernation. The muscles are said to be in a state of shock. This can lead to shortness of breath. The insufficient oxygen supply to the brain can cause dizziness and loss of consciousness.

Intense emotions including stress have been associated with an heart attack. Catecholamines are hormones produced by the adrenal gland. Epinephrine or adrenaline, which causes the fight or flight response

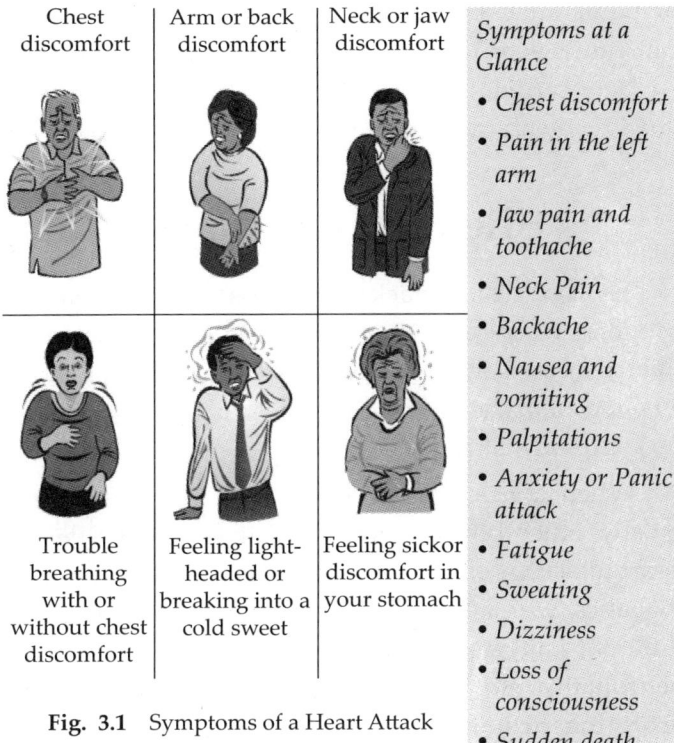

Fig. 3.1 Symptoms of a Heart Attack

Symptoms at a Glance

- *Chest discomfort*
- *Pain in the left arm*
- *Jaw pain and toothache*
- *Neck Pain*
- *Backache*
- *Nausea and vomiting*
- *Palpitations*
- *Anxiety or Panic attack*
- *Fatigue*
- *Sweating*
- *Dizziness*
- *Loss of consciousness*
- *Sudden death*

is one catecholamine. It can increase the heart rate, cardiac output and may even increase blood pressure. When the heart muscles are under so much stress, the sympathetic nervous system releases huge amount of catecholamines in the blood. They can cause nausea, vomiting, profuse sweating, palpitations and anxiety or panic attacks. Very high levels of catecholamines can cause ventricular arrhythmias and could lead to sudden cardiac arrest. When unable to resuscitate quickly, death can occurs minutes of cardiac arrest.

Silent Heart Attack

Most of heart attack symptoms start slowly and progress with exertion or time. It is also possible for them to occur suddenly and with great intensity. About 40 per cent of the patients who have heart attacks have no symptoms at all.

When a heart attack does not cause chest pain or any other typical symptoms, it is called a silent heart attack. A silent heart attack is more common in diabetics, women and elderly. Diabetics tend to have different pain thresholds and their chances of having neuropathy are high. People who have undergone heart transplant may not feel chest pain during a heart attack. In this case however, the patient's nerves are not connected to the transplanted heart.

In the Emergency Room

Since heart attack symptoms are sometimes obscure and do not always occur with chest pain, they are neglected. However, even the atypical symptoms are significant. It is crucial to get medical help immediately when one suspects a heart attack. It is best to avoid driving and ask for help. If you cannot find someone to drive you to the emergency room, call for an ambulance. If you are alone, remember to leave the main door unlocked.

Aspirin, a blood thinner, can help to restore some blood flow through the blocked arteries. Crush two aspirins, dissolve in a glass of water and take it immediately. If unable to crush them, chew them well and then swallow. Crushing the aspirin will allow it to be absorbed by the body faster than if it were just swallowed.

People with known coronary artery disease may be prescribed nitroglycerin for angina.

You can take it as directed under the tongue during a heart attack.

The aim of the medical professionals treating a heart attack would be to:

- Resume blood flow to the myocardium as soon as possible
- Provide supportive care to relieve pain and other symptoms
- To prevent further complications

Once in the emergency room, there will be swift activities trying to diagnose and treat without delay. Vital signs such as pulse, temperature, blood pressure and respiratory rate will be checked. You will be connected to a continuous blood pressure monitor. An electrocardiogram will confirm the story of a heart attack. It can even tell how many arteries are involved. Any irregular heartbeats or arrhythmias also can be found. An intravenous (IV) line will be inserted. Several blood tests will be done.

Supportive care including oxygen supplementation and pain medications will be given.

Beta blockers will be given to make the heart beat more forcefully yet slowly. This way the oxygen demand of the heart muscles are reduced a little. Several other medications depending on the symptoms and vital signs will be given.

The most important treatment is promptly injecting thrombolytic agents. Thrombolytic means clot dissolving. Blood clot occluding the coronary artery will start dissolving and the blood flow to the heart muscles can be restored. Early restoration implies lesser myocardial damage. Thrombolytic agents cannot be administered if you have a bleeding problem or have had a recent stroke. Some other reasons why this drug may not be administered are renal insufficiency, diabetic retinopathy and recent surgery.

Primary angioplasty is another method that can restore coronary artery blood flow in patients after a heart attack. Angioplasty is an invasive procedure where a thin tube called catheter is inserted into the blocked coronary artery through an artery in the groin or arm. There is a balloon at the end of this catheter. When the blockage is reached, the balloon is inflated, the plaque is compressed and the blood flow is restored. A small wire mesh tube called stent can be placed in the coronary artery to keep it open. If other revascularisation methods fail, emergency bypass surgery may be needed.

You must understand that the hospital experience varies from person to person and hospital to hospital. Treatments will be tailored to the patient's need or the availability of resources in the hospital. People who had heart attacks with no complications may be requested to stay in the Intensive care unit (ICU) or Coronary Care Unit (CCU) for a few days and then stepped down to normal hospital floors. They will be under observation, given rehabilitation and counselled to lead a better life. People with complications may require longer hospital stay.

Chapter 4
50 Causes of a Heart Attack

Modifiable Risk Factors

Atherosclerosis is considered as the main cause of coronary artery disease. However, there are several contributors or risk factors that increase a person's chance of having a heart attack. While some contributing factors cannot be changed, most of these risk factors can be either treated or prevented. By understanding these modifiable causes, you can lead your life defensively and lower the possibility of having a heart attack. After surviving a heart attack, it becomes much more important to keep these risk factors as low as possible.

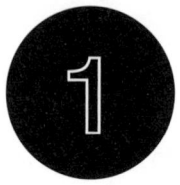

Smoking

The ill-effects of tobacco have been known for several decades. Yet, when asked if smoking is a major cause of heart disease in a survey, over 45 per cent of smokers answered no. We wouldn't be discussing smoking now if they were correct. Smoking doubles the risk of developing heart disease. The chance of sudden cardiac death in smokers with existing coronary artery disease is as high as 70 per cent.

Cigarettes contain thousands of chemicals in them, of which hundreds of them are toxic and carcinogenic. As you inhale, the chemicals reach your lungs and enter your bloodstream quickly. So, every single organ in your body receives these toxins. Even small levels of these chemicals can lead to inflammation of walls of the blood vessels or can narrow your blood vessels. Smoking causes atherosclerosis which hinders the blood flow through the arteries. The toxins in tobacco can modify the blood to clot more easily, thereby causing heart attacks or strokes. They can also cause peripheral artery disease and abdominal aortic aneurysms. They can cause cancer, several lung diseases, reduce fertility, miscarriages and even affect foetal development. They weaken your immune system and make you prone to recurrent infections. It increases the chances of developing diabetes and dyslipidemia. The risks are higher when the person who smokes has hypertension or high cholesterol levels.

> I only smoke one pack of cigarette a week. Am I safe? No.

There are no safe levels in smoking. Even if you had an occasional cigarette or even exposed to second-hand smokes, it is harmful. Second-hand smoking, also known as passive smoking, increases the risk of heart disease by about 30 per cent. The risk is higher for people who already have heart disease. Risks of developing diseases and its severity are high if:

- You started smoking early
- You are smoking heavily
- You've been smoking for several years
- You inhale the smokes deeply

Cigarettes have toxins such as nicotine, carbon monoxide and hydrogen cyanide that are addictive. The addictive components create receptors in the brain and keep you craving for more. People get attached to it biologically and psychologically. Teenagers get addicted more easily than adults.

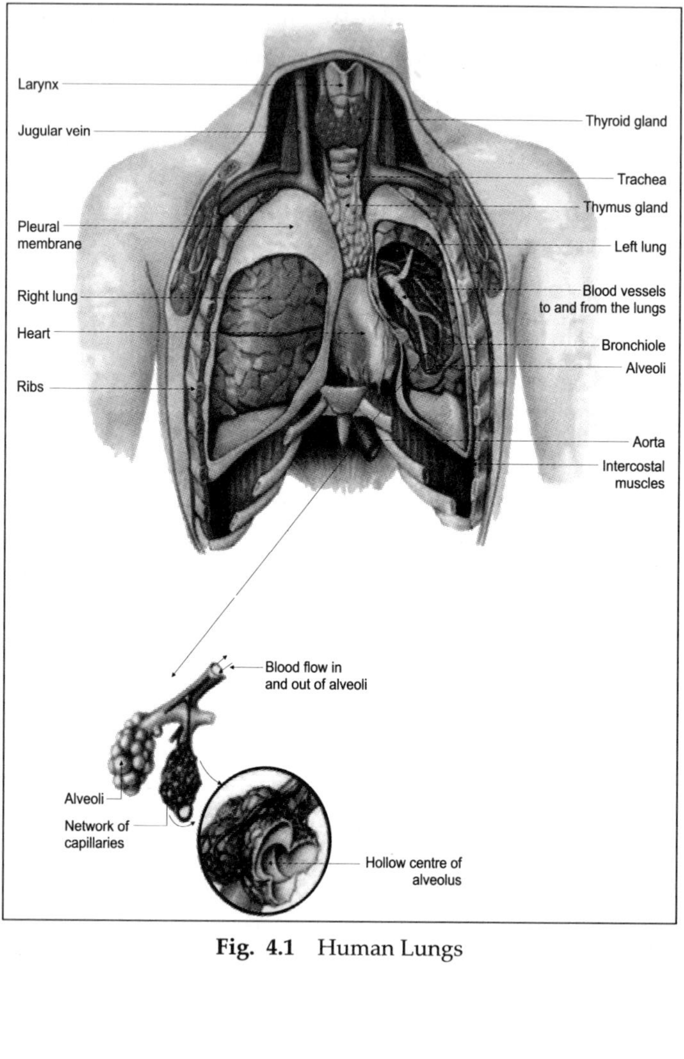

Fig. 4.1 Human Lungs

> I have switched to filtered cigarettes from regular cigarettes. Does that reduce the toxins entering my body? No.

Light, low nicotine or filtered cigarettes do not decrease the overall risks for developing diseases from tobacco. When you quit smoking, the risk of developing a heart attack reduces sharply in just one year. Death and several chronic disorders are preventable when you have never smoked or quit smoking immediately. It is never too late to quit smoking and the sooner, the better.

Hypertension

Systemic blood pressure (BP) is the pressure that blood pumped from the heart exerts upon the artery walls. Blood pressure is measured as systolic pressure over diastolic pressure in millimetres of mercury. For instance, a blood pressure reading can be 120/80 mmHg. Systolic blood pressure is the pressure when the heart is contracting, while diastolic blood pressure when the heart is relaxing.

Hypertension means high blood pressure. Hypotension means low blood pressure.

Table 4.1 Blood Pressure Chart

	Systolic pressure [Top number]	Diastolic number [Bottom number]
Normal BP	Less than 120	Less than 80
Pre hypertension	120 to 139	80 to 89
Stage I hypertension	140 to 159	90 to 99
Stage II hypertension	160 or more	100 or more
Hypotension	Less than 90	Less than 60

Hypertension can be easily diagnosed during a routine doctor visit. Over 90 per cent of the people with hypertension have not been associated with any medical condition leading to the rise in blood pressure, while about 10 per cent of them have some diseases in the kidney, arteries or endocrine system. Certain medications can also increase the blood pressure.

Typically, blood pressure increases with age and tends to run in the family. Other reasons that can put you at risk for high blood pressure are smoking, obesity, sedentary lifestyle, increased salt intake in diet, stress, drinking too much alcohol and sleep apnoea.

Hypertension may not cause any symptoms for years. But persistent high blood pressure can be a major risk factor for heart attack, heart failure, stroke, aneurysms, renal impairment, retinopathy and some times, even vision loss.

Hypertension and the Heart

Hypertension causes several diseases of the heart such as rhythm abnormalities, valve diseases, heart failure, decreased blood supply to the myocardium and heart attacks and also affects the size and thickness of the heart chambers.

The heart has to pump extra hard against the elevated pressure in the arteries. The increase in work load weakens the heart muscles. Shear stress caused by high blood pressure on the arterial wall damages its endothelial lining. This accelerates the accumulation of plaque in the coronary arteries and can result in a heart attack. If you are over forty years of age, blood pressure increase by every 20mmHg of systolic and 10mmHg of diastolic can double your risk of heart disease.

If hypertension is diagnosed at an early stage, treatment can be done with lifestyle modifications such as reducing salt intake, losing weight, quitting smoking, reducing alcohol intake, managing stress and treating sleep apnoea. Medications will be added only if these changes are not enough to bring the blood pressure back to normal.

Dyslipidemia

The discovery of cholesterol in atherosclerotic plaques was made over a hundred years ago. Since then, the theory that reducing cholesterol in blood would reduce coronary artery disease exists. The term 'lipid' refers to all classes of fats and fat-like substances in the blood. A lipid panel blood test commonly measures the amount of total cholesterol, triglycerides, high-density lipoprotein (HDL), low-density lipoprotein (LDL) and very low-density lipoprotein (VLDL).

Lipid disorders can be inherited. Some genetic changes may cause excessive production or less clearing of cholesterol in the body. The secondary causes are diabetes, excessive alcohol intake, kidney disease, cirrhosis, hypothyroidism and several medications.

Cholesterol does not dissolve in blood. In order for it to be transported in the body, it uses carriers called lipoproteins. LDL (also known as bad cholesterol) can transport cholesterol into the walls of the arteries and start the plaque formation in coronary arteries, carotid arteries and peripheral arteries. HDL cholesterol (also known as good cholesterol) carries the extra cholesterol from the arteries back to the liver to be excreted.

Triglycerides are fats that come from the diet you eat. It circulates in the blood especially after a high-fat or high-sugar meal. Excess triglycerides become fatty deposits in the blood vessels increasing the risk of cardiovascular diseases. High triglyceride levels are also passed on genetically; they may also be found in people with diabetes, hypothyroidism and obesity.

Desired levels of Lipids [milligrams/decilitre]

Cholesterol – Less than 200 mg/dl

Triglycerides – Less than 150 mg/dl

LDL – Less than 100mg/dl

HDL – Greater than 50mg/dl

Treating lipid disorders with medications will aim to decrease LDL and triglyceride levels. Regular aerobic exercise can help increase HDL levels. Reducing weight, quitting cigarettes and eating healthy can also help to maintain normal lipid levels.

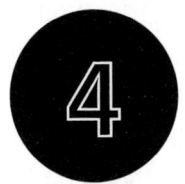# Diabetes

Diabetes mellitus or diabetes is a condition where the blood sugar level is higher than normal. Insulin is a hormone that is secreted by the pancreas which regulates the sugar level in blood. Diabetes is divided into three types.

Type I or insulin-dependant diabetes mellitus is a condition where a person's body does not produce enough insulin.

Type II or non-insulin dependant diabetes mellitus is a condition where the insulin produced is not being properly utilised.

Gestational diabetes is a condition where a pregnant woman has high blood sugar levels. She is not a diabetic before pregnancy and has a very high chance of developing Type II diabetes later.

A fasting blood glucose test is done in the morning before breakfast. The normal range is usually about 70 to 100mg/dl. Postprandial blood glucose is done two hours after a meal and the normal range is less than 140mg/dl. Hyperglycaemia is a state where the blood sugar levels are higher than normal. Hypoglycaemia is a state where the blood sugar level is below 60mg/dl.

Few causes of diabetes are hereditary, age, obesity, poor diet, stress, sedentary lifestyle, dyslipidemia and some medications. Uncontrolled diabetes may lead to diabetes retinopathy, renal impairment, neuropathy and heart disease.

If you are a diabetic, your chance of getting heart disease or stroke is 50 per cent more than non-diabetics. More than 80 per cent of the diabetics die because of some form of heart disease. Atherosclerotic coronary artery disease is the most common form of heart disease in diabetics. They tend to have low HDL and high triglyceride levels which increase the risk of atherosclerosis. The risk is increased threefold in diabetics who smoke, have high blood pressure or are overweight.

Diabetics who have heart attacks have double the chances of dying when compared to non-diabetics. Hence, it is very important for them to keep the sugar levels near normal and be closely monitored and treated by their doctors.

Haemoglobin A1c (HbA1c) is a small component of haemoglobin that has glucose bound to it. It is also known as glycosylated haemoglobin. The level of HbA1c in blood depends on the amount of sugar

Diabetes: Complication

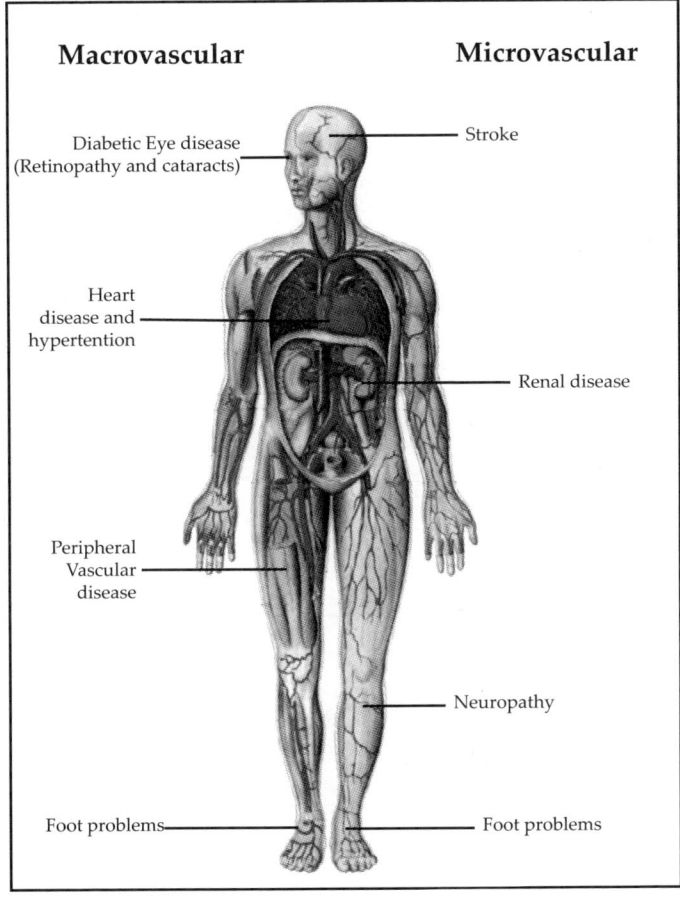

Fig. 4.2 Complications of Diabetes

concentrated in blood. A blood test to check HbA1c level can indicate the average level of sugar in blood for the past 2-3 months. Normal value of HbA1c is less than 6 per cent. Diabetics should keep it less than 7 per cent to prevent or delay complications caused by diabetics. This test may be ordered by your doctor every three months along with fasting and postprandial blood sugars to see how well your diabetes is under control.

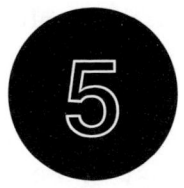

Thyroid Imbalance

The thyroid gland is a small gland located in the neck that produces thyroid hormone. This hormone is essential to regulate many vital functions and metabolisms of the body. The thyroid hormone affects almost every cell in the body and also increases the basal metabolic rate.

Hypothyroidism is a condition where the thyroid gland does not produce enough thyroid hormone. Hyperthyroidism is a condition where the thyroid gland produces excess hormones. Both these conditions are not uncommon and have a great effect on the heart.

Less thyroid hormone can weaken the heart muscles and hamper its effective pumping. So, the amount of blood that is pumped out of the heart with each beat is reduced. The amount of blood reaching the myocardium is also reduced. It can accelerate and worsen the already existing coronary artery disease by increasing LDL cholesterol and C-reactive protein levels. Moreover, hypothyroidism can cause the blood vessels to stiffen and cause further obstruction to the blood flowing in those arteries resulting in a heart attack.

Studies show that women with this condition have very high chances of having hardened aortas and are twice likely to have a heart attack. Hypothyroidism may also lead to heart failure. Other cardiac effects are low heart rate and low blood pressure.

Other symptoms of hypothyroidism are depression, fatigue, muscle aches, weight gain, hair loss and joint pains.

In hyperthyroidism, the heart rate is increased along with its force of contraction. The oxygen demand of the heart muscles is increased greatly. People may have abnormally fast heart rhythm and high blood pressure. The heart gets tired after working hard for a long time and can result in heart failure. People with existing coronary artery disease may find that their angina and other symptoms are worsening and may even have a heart attack.

Blood tests can show the amount of thyroid hormones in blood. Thyroid supplementation may be given to treat hypothyroidism. Radioactive iodine may also be used to treat hyperthyroidism.

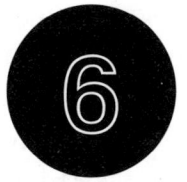

Obesity

Being overweight may start as a cosmetic problem for many. If you are obese, you might endure snide remarks and jokes about your appearance from friends, family or even complete strangers. Low self-esteem may not be the only drawback of being overweight or obese. Your weight has a direct impact on your health. Obesity increases your chances of getting diabetes or hypertension by three times or more, which further contributes to heart diseases. There is an increased risk of getting cancer. Although being overweight does not mean that you will die of heart disease, the risks of developing coronary artery disease are high.

There is a difference between being overweight and obese. Body mass index (BMI) or Quetelet index is used to estimate a healthy body weight based on a person's height. A simple formula to measure BMI is weight in kilograms divided by the square of height in meters.

$$BMI = \frac{\text{Weight (Kg)}}{(\text{Height (m)})^2}$$

Healthy BMI is 19 to 24. BMI from 25-29 signifies overweight and BMI over 30 indicates obesity.

Another form of obesity that is the strongest risk factor for heart disease is abdominal obesity. Central obesity or belly fat strongly increases the risk for heart diseases. Studies show that the ratio of the waist size to the hip size should be 1:1 in men and 0.8:1 in women.

Since being overweight increases the chances of having heart attacks, it is important to maintain a healthy weight or take proper steps to lose weight.

A major problem that is now gripping the whole world is childhood obesity. Being overweight used to be an issue mostly faced by adults only. Over the past few decades, the prevalence of morbid obesity in children and teenagers is drastically increasing. Improper diet, less physical activity and genes are the main contributing factors for these children to gain excess weight. They are at the risk of developing bone and joint problems and sleep disturbances. They are also at great risk of onset of adult diseases such as Type II diabetes, stroke, cancer and heart diseases at a very early age. Being overweight can impede their day-to-day activities and cause social and psychological problems.

Parents, teachers and medical professionals must contribute equally to help such children get back in shape. Steps must be taken to prevent childhood obesity to create a healthier future.

Chilhood Obesity Complications

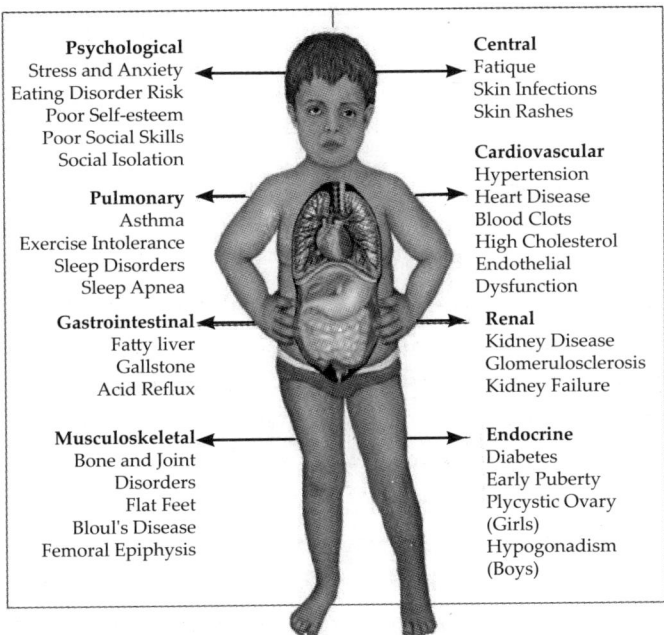

Fig. 4.3 Complications of Childhood Obesity

Sedentary Lifestyle

Sedentary lifestyle means physical inactivity or lack of regular exercise. It is one of the major preventable causes of heart diseases. Unlike many other risk factors, physical inactivity is commonly a choice that you make with or without understanding its consequences. You have a sedentary lifestyle if you are sitting down most of the day, have an inactive job and do not exercise at least 30 minutes everyday.

Regular aerobic exercise helps your heart and lungs work well. Your muscles use oxygen efficiently. With inactive lifestyle, your body becomes tired more easily and you feel short of breath with just walking a short distance. With long standing inactivity, your body's ability to do physical activities declines. You lose flexibility, strength and effort tolerance.

The chances of having fatal heart attacks are doubled with a sedentary lifestyle. You are more prone to develop diabetes, obesity, hypertension, depression, dyslipidemia and bone problems. Your immune system is weakened and you are more prone to infections.

Choosing an active lifestyle over inactivity has plenty of benefits. It can help lower weight and blood pressure. It can increase HDL cholesterol levels. It helps reduce stress and depression. It can improve joint function and reduce fatigue. Overall, even moderate amounts of exercise have positive impact on health and should not be neglected.

Alcohol

People often question if drinking is right or wrong. There are several studies that indicate drinking in moderation is good for your heart. So, how much is the right amount? The American Heart Association says one or two drinks per day for men and one drink for women. Red wine has antioxidants such as flavonoids and other anti-clotting properties that help reduce the risk of heart disease. Moderate amount of alcohol has been known to improve the levels of HDL (good cholesterol).

But drinking excess alcohol leads to high blood pressure, obesity, alcoholism, dyslipidemia, stroke and accidents. Alcoholism has destroyed many lives. Although not everyone who drinks is an alcoholic, there is no way to predict who would get more influenced by it. Alcohol is very addictive and even very small amounts may not be safe to a few who cannot tolerate it well. Some find it very hard to control the amount they drink once they start drinking regularly.

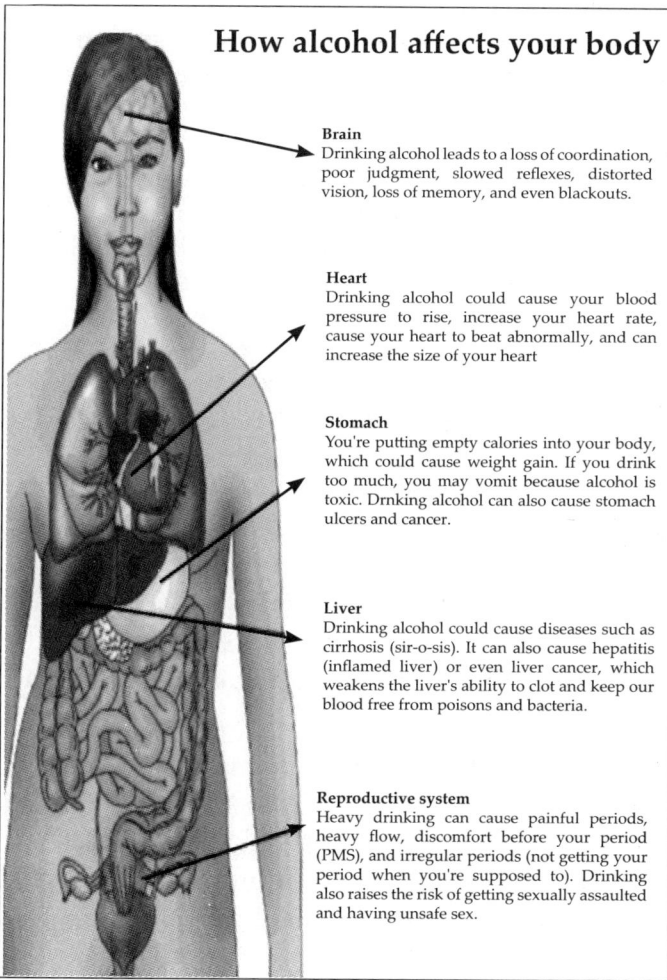

Fig. 4.5 Ill-effects of Excessive Alcohol on the Body

Men and women metabolise alcohol in different ways. Your body metabolises alcohol in a less effective way as you get older. People who have uncontrolled hypertension, dyslipidemia, pancreatitis, liver disease, heart failure or a history of alcoholism should restrain from drinking alcohol. Pregnant women should not drink. Since alcohol can interfere in blood clotting mechanism, people who regularly take antiplatelet medications such as aspirin or plavix should consult their doctor before drinking.

Effects on the heart

Excess alcohol has a straight toxic effect on the heart. In due course, heavy drinking causes high blood pressure, cardiomyopathy and heart failure. Heavy drinking increases the level of cholesterol and triglycerides in blood, thereby increasing the risk for heart attacks. Binge drinking can worsen heart disease and double the risk of heart attacks.

Although little alcohol is beneficial for the heart, a little more than recommended is dangerous. Hence, doctors do not recommend people who refrain from alcohol to start drinking just to improve their health. Instead, they encourage them to eat healthy and exercise everyday.

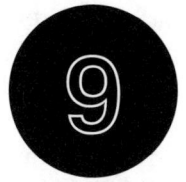# Diet

Diet plays a vital role for a healthy heart. Depending on the type of food, it can either reduce or increase your risk for heart disease. For example, if you eat a diet that is high in fat and sodium, you may be highly contributing a lot to coronary artery disease.

Food that has high amount of saturated fat increases cholesterol level in blood. Cholesterol accumulates in the arteries and starts to clog arteries. This is the beginning of coronary artery disease. When people with heart disease continue to eat saturated fat, their risk of heart attack is high.

Fat intake should be less than 35 per cent of your total daily calories. Examples of foods that contain a lot of saturated fats are whole milk, ice cream, butter, lard, bacon, coconut and palm oils. Trans fats are seen usually in processed foods. They raise the levels of LDL cholesterol and decrease HDL cholesterol. This imbalance in cholesterol can also lead to heart disease.

The amount of food that you eat everyday also matters. When you eat more food than required, your daily caloric intake increases. This can lead to obesity and diabetes doubling the chances of a heart attack.

High salt intake increases blood pressure. Hypertension is a leading risk factor for strokes and heart attacks. By lowering the salt intake in your diet, you can reduce your blood pressure and maintain a healthier heart.

Sleep Apnoea

The word 'apnoea' means without breath. If you have sleep apnoea, then you stop breathing during your sleep over and over again. There are three types of sleep apnoea – central; obstructive; and mixed. Central sleep apnoea is a condition where the brain does not signal the muscles to breathe. Obstructive sleep apnoea means that the air passage is blocked when the soft tissues in the throat collapses during sleep. Mixed sleep apnoea is a combination of the other two conditions.

Apnoea can occur at any age, but is more common in adults. Being overweight increases the chances of one having obstructive sleep apnoea. Problems associated with untreated sleep apnoea are hypertension, memory loss, irritability, fatigue and headaches. Abnormal heart rhythm, increased risk for stroke and sudden death are some serious complications of sleep apnoea.

Sleep apnoea acts as a trigger for heart attacks at night. Sleep apnoea increases the amount of adrenaline causing a rise in blood pressure and reduces the amount of oxygen that is pumped to the heart. Repeated episodes of sleep apnoea can starve the heart muscles and result in a heart attack.

Most people do not realise they have sleep apnoea. But it can be easily diagnosed and treated effectively.

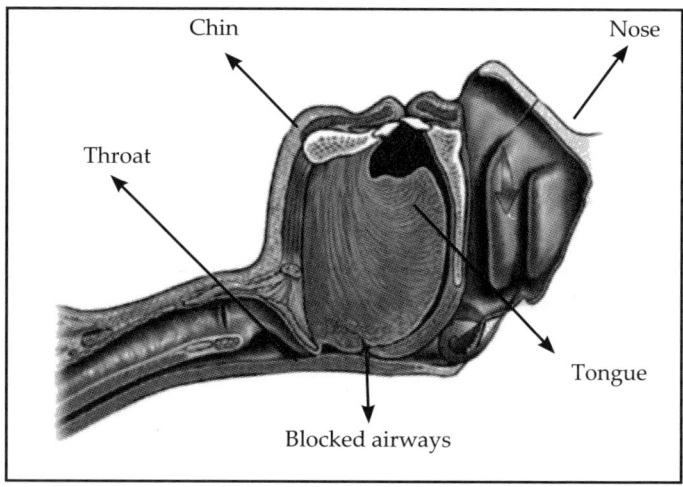

Fig. 4.6 Airway Obstruction in Sleep Apnoea

 # Mental Stress

Human body responds to numerous physical and psychological demands by making changes that are hard and undesirable. Also, stress can be caused due to emotional, mental and behavioural demands. For some, stress is the feeling that they are stretched to their limits and they are about to burst like a balloon.

Everybody experiences stress from time to time and not all of it is detrimental. Hans Selye, an endocrinologist, coined the word 'Eustress' which defines healthy stress. For example, during recreational sports, you may experience happiness or a feeling of exhilaration, which is healthy. The stress that harms your body is often associated with feelings of distress such as anger, fatigue, frustration and anxiety.

The body's response to stress often produces a 'fight or flight response'. A lot of chemicals are released in the body and the heart begins to beat faster, the blood pressure rises and pre-blood is pumped to muscles that needs to respond. To provide the body with more energy, fat from the stored tissues are transformed into fatty acids. These responses are often helpful in dangerous situations, like for instance, when someone is getting mugged or caught in fire, the rush of adrenaline can lead them to safety.

Mental and emotional stresses are different from physical stresses. The response to mental and emotional stress can be injurious to health. Unlike a physical stress situation, the hormones and fat released during mental stress are not used up by the muscles. Heart rate and blood pressure remains high and the unnecessary tension damages walls of the arteries. Repeated stress situations causes atherosclerosis and over time, repeated stress speeds up coronary artery blockage. While stress hormones cause healthy arteries to dilate and allow more blood through it, it constricts a diseased artery. This can cause a coronary artery to close off completely, resulting in a heart attack.

Some symptoms of excessive stress are:
- Being tearful
- Irritable
- Unusual body aches
- Drnking or smoking more than usual
- Insomnia
- Reduced appetite
- Fatigue
- Less concentration

Identifying the source of stress and dealing with it is one good way of handling stress. Drnking plenty of water, regular exercise and a healthy diet can help reduce anxiety and stress. Slow deep breathing, talking to friends and a stress management class can also help reduce stress in life.

Emotional Disorders

Heart disease is more than just a physical illness. Getting diagnosed with heart disease can cause emotional and psychological distress. Likewise, the emotional and psychological distress can contribute to myocardial infarctions and strokes.

Intense negative emotions may trigger spasm of the coronary arteries and rupture of the blockage in the arteries. It is also associated with increased aggregation of platelets. All these can lead to a major heart attack.

Anger

When doctors observed that patients with heart disease seemed agitated, frustrated, unable to relax and angry, they decided to study the connection between different behaviours and coronary artery disease. Cardiologists Meyer Friedman and R.H. Rosenman described Type A behaviour as a risk factor for coronary artery disease. A person with Type A personality is one who is aggressive, compulsive, competitive and unable to accept things that do not go as planned. A person with Type B personality is one who is relaxed, laid back and less aggressive. Some studies comparing the two types showed that people with Type A behaviour had more incidence of coronary artery disease and the extent of the disease was also high. Some studies have failed to prove that anger and hostility causes coronary heart disease, though it seemed to worsen the condition of the existing coronary artery disease.

Depression

A large number of people diagnosed with coronary artery disease have significant depression. Depression is often increased with an episode of heart attack or after bypass surgery and may last for several months. Depression poses several problems in heart patients because it worsens their symptoms and their prognosis. Depression often prevents patients from an angioplasty or heart surgery. When you are depressed, you are less likely to exercise, comply with medical treatment and return to your regular activities soon. You may resort to excess food, alcohol or cigarettes every time you feel unhappy.

Depression is more common in women and diabetics. It is an established risk factor for healthy individuals to develop coronary artery disease. The risk increases with the severity of depression. After a heart attack, depression leads to a poor quality of life, increases the chances of a recurrent attack, arrhythmias and even death.

A person who has Type D personality is always gloomy, irritable and worried. Type D people have increased negative emotions and have social inhibitions. Research has shown that their prognosis after a heart attack is worse when compared to a person with non- Type D personality. Their risk of another attack and death is very high.

Anxiety

Chronic anxiety or panic attacks can initiate or accelerate the progress of coronary artery disease. It also increases the risk of mortality. There is at least a two-fold increased risk of recurrent heart attack, arrhythmias and sudden cardiac death in patients with severe anxiety. This may be because anxiety increases the production of catecholamines and decreases the amount of blood flowing through the arteries.

Other negative factors such as mistrust or cynicism may also contribute to coronary artery disease.

Poor Dental Health

A bright white smile and a fresh breath are great, not just for your appearance and confidence, but also for your overall well-being. Who could imagine that good oral health increases your lifespan? Healthy gums and teeth causes less tooth fall. Adults look a lot younger with all their teeth intact than showing gaps.

Gum disease initially starts as bleeding, swollen or tender gums. If not taken care of, this condition worsens with time and leads to tooth loss. It sounds unlikely and is hard to believe that a problem that starts in your mouth can hurt your body elsewhere. Cavities and gum disease do not just cause a toothache, but they can also lead to chest pain.

Researches found that gum diseases increase the chances of having a heart attack by 25 per cent. The bacteria from periodontal diseases were found in the plaques that blocks the coronary arteries. There are millions of bacteria surviving in your mouth. Unless your teeth are well-maintained, these bacteria enter the blood vessels. The immune system gets stressed and in response, causes narrowing of the arteries or inflammation. Also, these micro-organisms attach themselves to the plaques in the arteries. This can lead to blood clot formations and increased blockages, thereby increasing the risk of heart attack and stroke.

Other diseases associated with gum disorders are sleep disorders, cancer, lung diseases such as pneumonia and metabolic syndromes like diabetes. It is important that pregnant women take good care of their oral heath to avoid delivering pre-term babies and miscarriages.

What can you do to avoid periodontal diseases?

- Brush atleast twice a day
- Floss as needed
- Visit your dentist atleast twice a year to get your teeth cleaned
- Eat a healthy diet
- Avoid carbonated beverages
- Avoid smoking as it can affect all the tissues in your mouth

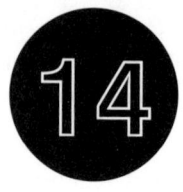

Hormone Replacement Therapy

Heart attacks in women are very different from those experienced by men. Most women have a silent attack or their symptoms are so vague that they do not relate it to the heart.

Absence of symptoms or plainly ignoring them puts them at a greater risk for death. The chances of women having a second heart attack are doubled when compared to men.

It is necessary to promptly investigate symptoms such as shortness of breath, unusual fatigue, indigestion, anxiety and sleep disturbances to prevent a heart attack. Women may also present with weakness, cold sweats or dizziness.

Heart disease happens more in older women than younger. This is because, at menopause, the oestrogen level is decreasing. Oestrogen relaxes the blood vessels and removes free radicals that can harm the arterial wall. Oestrogen is associated with low levels of bad cholesterol and high levels of good cholesterol, thereby preventing atherosclerosis. After menopause, the balance between the cholesterol is lost along with lowering oestrogen levels. To prevent complications such as osteoporosis or coronary artery disease, hormone replacement therapy (HRT) was started a few years ago.

However, recent studies on long term hormone replacement have shown that the potential health benefits may not be completely true. Though HRT provides some benefits, there were risks such as increased blood clotting, due to which new guidelines were formed to prevent complications from using hormone replacements. HRT is not used for preventing heart attacks and strokes, and long term use is not recommended as it can increase the risk of heart attacks, strokes and breast cancer.

One other factor that may contribute to cardiovascular diseases in women is oral birth control pills. However, the studies have shown conflicting results regarding this. Women on birth control pills and smoke, or over the age of 35, are at an increased risk of having a heart attack. It is necessary to make sure that there are no pre-existing risks for heart disease before starting oral contraceptives.

Non-Modifiable Risk Factors

There are three major risk factors for heart attacks that you cannot eliminate or change. These non-modifiable risk factors are age, sex and having a family history of heart disease. Although these risk factors cannot be changed, keeping the modifiable risk factors away may keep you from having a heart attack.

Age

Coronary artery disease is a degenerative disease. So, it is more likely to occur as you get old. Being over 45 years of age for men and 55 for women is considered a risk factor. Majority of the patients with a heart attack are over 65 years of age. Women after menopause carry the same amount of risk as men their age.

Each person ages differently and the rate at which changes occur to their cardiovascular function vary. As you get older, the arteries lose its elasticity and stiffen. This raises blood pressure. The heart walls may thicken and decrease its strength of contraction. So, the heart may not pump blood efficiently as it did before. The blood and oxygen supplied to muscles including myocardium is less.

The outcome after a heart attack in elderly patients is poor. The capacity of producing new heart cells after apoptosis is reduced and further leads to dysfunction of the heart. They do not respond well to adrenaline as well as young people, so their responses to stress or disease may add harm to coronary arteries.

Heart attacks can occur in people under 40 years of age if they have some other major contributing factor like smoking or uncontrolled hypertension. Habits such as eating fatty foods or sedentary lifestyle that cause atherosclerosis start as early as childhood. People have to realise these habits will cause huge health problems and start controlling them as soon as possible. Asymptomatic men under 45 with other risk factors for coronary artery disease should get screening tests done to prevent heart attacks.

Sex

In the past, heart disease was considered a man's disease. However, heart does not show any favouritism to women. The only difference is heart disease starts a little later in a woman's life, after her menopause. But this does not buy younger women immunity if they have other risk factors such as hypertension or smoking. Oestrogen in women may offer some protection to women before menopause. Once the oestrogen levels decrease in the body, a woman's probability of having a heart attack is same as that of a man. Smoking reduces the oestrogen level in women and definitely puts them at a greater risk for heart attacks even at a young age.

Symptoms experienced by men and women during a heart attack are quite different. While most men experience acute chest pain or pain in the arm, women may have non-specific symptoms like indigestion and fatigue. This may prevent or delay prompt diagnosis and result in severe complications, including death.

Heart disease is the main cause of death in both men and women, but more fatal heart attacks are seen in women. The number of women dying from a heart attack is way higher than women dying from breast cancer.

There are ongoing researches on coronary artery diseases and women now, to see how prevention and treatment plans vary between men and women.

Hereditary

You may be a person who eats healthy, exercises, does not smoke or even drink alcohol. Unfortunately, you've been diagnosed with heart disease. Your genetic predisposition to this disease may be the culprit here and you can hardly do anything to change your family history. But look on the bright side; at least you did not choose to smoke or drink heavily. This could have caused a deadly heart attack at a younger age.

The outlook of the disease changes when a close family member has premature heart disease. For those people along with lifestyle modifications, medications may become necessary. If your mother, father or a sibling died of a heart attack under the age of sixty, your risk is above average when compared to someone who does not have this family history. Almost 80 per cent of the people who are diagnosed with heart disease under the age of 60 have genes that contribute to atherosclerosis.

Your family has a strong influence in your upbringing. Your childhood environment makes a big contribution to your modifiable risk factors. If your parents smoked at home, you were exposed to secondary smokes and you are more prone to be a smoker. If they ate too much fried foods, they probably fed you the same.

You can also be genetically predisposed to other contributing risk factors such as diabetes, high cholesterol and hypertension. There may be a day in the future when scientists find a way to go about correcting these genes. Until then, you have to do the best you can to keep these risk factors in control. That is the positive aspect of knowing your background which gives you an extra motivation to develop healthier habits.

Coronary Artery Disease/Injury

Coronary arteries are the arteries that supply blood and oxygen to the heart. When these arteries become diseased and damaged the heart muscles are deprived of oxygen. This is called myocardial ischemia. Ischemia may present itself as angina (chest pain). When the damage increases, some part of the muscles die because of oxygen starvation. This causes a heart attack. The most common cause of coronary artery is due to atherosclerosis or narrowing of the artery by fatty deposits. There are few other causes that can cause sudden narrowing of the coronary arteries. They are coronary spasm, certain congenital heart diseases, thrombus in the coronary artery and dissection. Rarely medical treatments or surgery can cause injury or narrowing of the coronary arteries.

 # Atherosclerosis

Normally arteries are strong, elastic and flexible with smooth layers on the inside that allows free blood flow. Atherosclerosis is a degenerative process where fatty materials start to accumulate in the inner wall of the arteries and the lumen becomes thick and irregular. In addition to the fat calcium deposits also add to the block and the plaque gets harder. As you get older the arteries become less elastic and thick. Injury to the artery wall can lead to scarring or attract more platelets and other coagulants to the site and increase the size of the plaque. Heart attack often occurs when this plaque ruptures and the thrombus causes a complete blockage of blood to the heart.

Fat accumulation starts in the second decade of life. But moderate to severe atherosclerosis normally starts later in life. Risk factors such as hypertension, smoking or diabetes that causes constant injury to the arteries can increase the progression of atherosclerosis. Symptoms of coronary artery disease start gradually. Atherosclerosis often presents as chest pain or angina and alerts you to take more care of your heart. But sometimes there may be no symptoms until a heart attack occurs.

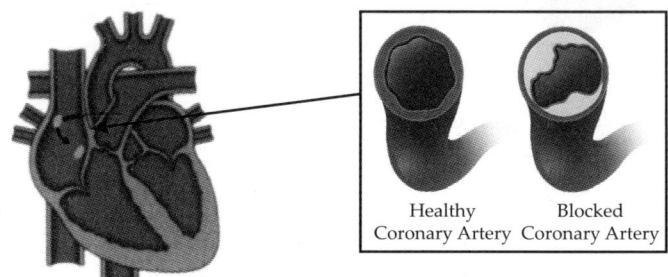

Fig. 4.8 Atherosclerosis

Although there is no complete cure for atherosclerosis, its progression can be slowed by lowering its risk factors with lifestyle changes and medications. When medications do not treat the symptoms adequately or if there is severe blockage, an angioplasty or coronary artery bypass surgery may be required.

Coronary Artery Spasm

Coronary artery spasm is another reason other than atherosclerosis that causes narrowing of a coronary artery. The muscle fibres around the coronary artery go into a sudden and temporary spasm that causes chest pain or heart attack. About 2 per cent people with angina have coronary artery spasm. It is also known as variant angina or Prinzmetal angina.

Most people with variant angina have coronary artery disease. In patients with atherosclerosis, chest pain occurs when the heart is exerted and the oxygen demand is not met. But coronary spasm often occurs at night while you are asleep and wakes you up. The spasm may even make you lose your consciousness. It is also triggered with exposure to cold, emotional stress, alcohol withdrawal, cigarette smoking, vasoconstrictors (medicines that causes blood vessel narrowing) and illegal drugs.

Nitroglycerin taken during an episode of variant angina can relieve the symptoms. Other medications to treat coronary artery disease can improve blood supply to the heart muscles. If the triggering factors are avoided, the chances of coronary artery spasm are low.

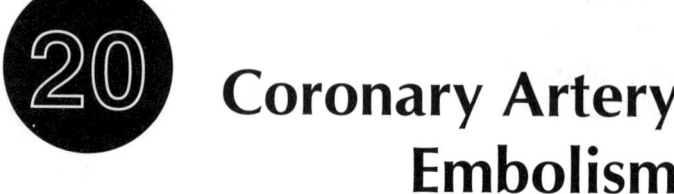

Coronary Artery Embolism

A blood clot in a blood vessel or in the heart is called a thombus. A thrombus that travels from one part of the body to block another artery or a vein is called an embolus. Atherosclerosis in the arteries is one reason for embolism. Other diseases that increase the chances of having an embolism are rheumatic heart disease, atrial fibrillation, mitral stenosis, prosthetic valves in the heart and infective endocarditis.

Coronary artery occlusion due to an embolus is a dramatic event and can cause a severe heart attack. Symptoms of an embolus can start slowly or very quickly depending on the size of the blood clot and the amount of blood it is restricting from flowing through the artery. During a heart attack a patient may feel chest pain, shortness of breath, palpitations, dizziness, nausea, vomiting and excessive sweating.

Mortality rate is high when emboli are not treated promptly. Thrombolytic agents are given intravenously to dissolve the clot. Anticoagulants such as heparin or warfarin are given to prevent clot formation in people with atrial fibrillation or mitral stenosis. Medications to treat coronary artery disease will be also given to prevent a heart attack.

Coronary Artery Dissection

Coronary artery dissection is a rare disease mainly affecting women. There is a tear in the coronary artery that causes the blood too flow through the tear. Dissection can be spontaneous or may be caused due to a catheter injury during an angiogram and trauma.

The main symptom of coronary dissection is a heart attack mostly followed by sudden cardiac death. Most women seem to develop it in pregnancy or post partum stage. Its aetiology is unknown. Another triggering factor may be hypertension.

Spontaneous coronary artery dissection is not a predictable disease and death is most often the first symptom. Some people with chronic dissection have been diagnosed with heart failure. Atherosclerosis has been associated with a few coronary artery dissection patients.

Coronary artery dissection should be suspected in a middle aged women presenting with heart attack and no risk factors for heart disease. Early angiogram may identify the presence of this condition. Angioplasty with stent placement or coronary artery bypass surgery may be required to treat this disease.

Diseases of the Heart and Arteries

When you hear the word heart disease, the first thing that comes to mind is coronary artery disease. There are several diseases of the heart and some of them can lead to a myocardial infarction. Cardiovascular disease is a very broad term. Cardio means heart and vascular means blood vessels. Structural or functional dysfunction of the heart and the blood vessels may impede proper blood flow to the myocardium and cause a heart attack.

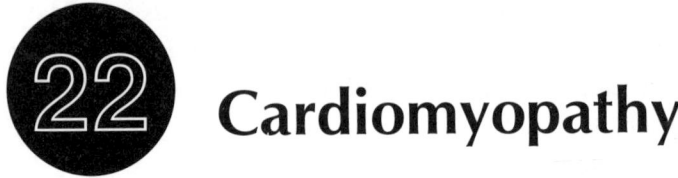

Cardiomyopathy

Cardiomyopathy is the disease of the heart muscle. Cardiomyopathy interferes with the heart's ability to pump blood out efficiently. Ischemic cardiomyopathy is when a heart attack or coronary artery disease causes cardiomyopathy and the other types are non-ischemic. Several things can cause cardiomyopathy and some of them are myocarditis, diabetes, alcohol, genetic, post partum and viral infections.

Cardiomyopathy is classified into dilated, hypertrophic and restrictive. In the dilated or congestive form, the heart walls are dilated and the muscles are weakened. The heart does not contract properly. Blood is pooled in the chambers and that can cause clot formation, which in turn results in stroke or heart attack. In the hypertrophic form, the heart muscles are thickened and are unable to contract properly. They can cause several fatal arrhythmias and some form of hypertrophic cardiomyopathy can obstruct the blood flowing through the heart. In the restrictive form, the heart does not fill adequately before contracting, so not enough blood is pumped out.

Most patients may have no symptoms at all. As the cardiomyopathy worsens, shortness of breath and fatigue can occur. Chest pain and dizziness are associated with some forms of cardiomyopathies. Asymptomatic patients may not require any treatment. Sometimes, treating the cause helps. For some, treatments may be directed towards treating their symptoms and reducing complications. Sometimes, surgery is needed to remove excess tissue obstructing blood flow or a heart transplant is needed as a last resort. Some others may require pacemaker and Implantable Cardioverter Defibrillator (ICD) implantation.

While some inherited forms cannot be prevented, you can reduce the possibility of having ischemic cardiomyopathy with a healthy lifestyle and taking care of other medical conditions that cause cardiomyopathy.

Heart Cancer

Normal cells in the human body divide and form new cells. Occasionally some cells divide abnormally and rapidly without control even when they are not supposed to. The abnormal cells clump together to form tumours. Malignant tumours are cancerous. They invade the tissues nearby and can even spread to other organs.

Cancer of the heart is extremely rare and most of us have never heard such a thing exists. Primary tumours are tumours that originate in the heart. Myxomas, fibromas and rhabdomyomas are forms of non-cancerous tumours of the heart. Sarcoma is the most common form of primary malignant heart tumour. Tumours that originate elsewhere in the body and then spread via metastasis to the heart are called secondary heart tumours. Though uncommon, secondary heart cancer is relatively more common than primary heart cancer.

Most often, the diagnosis of cardiac sarcoma is overlooked because they are rare and the signs and symptoms are non-specific. They may present with chest pain, fatigue or shortness of breath. Heart cancer may not be discovered during a regular physical examination. The incidence of heart tumours including benign tumours is less than 0.02 per cent; they can occur at any age in both men and women.

Electrocardiogram (ECG) and Chest X-ray may have non-specific abnormalities. Echocardiogram and CT scan can help detecting these lesions. MRI can define its proper location and its damage to the surrounding structures.

Malignant tumours of the heart spread rapidly, so majority of patients have metastasis when they have symptoms. The tumours can be found in any chambers of the heart or on its wall. The symptoms depend on the location of the tumour and the extent of metastasis. The heart tumours can obstruct blood flow and proper valve function. When the blood flowing through the coronary arteries is reduced, it results in a heart attack. They can also cause arrhythmias and pericardia effusion. Other symptoms associated with heart cancer are heart failure, fever, embolism and anaemia.

Few methods to treat heart cancer are chemotherapy, radiation, surgical excision and heart transplant. Prognosis is better if heart cancer is treated by surgical removal, but not all tumours can be completely excised. Partial excision may be performed to improve symptoms or for biopsy purposes.

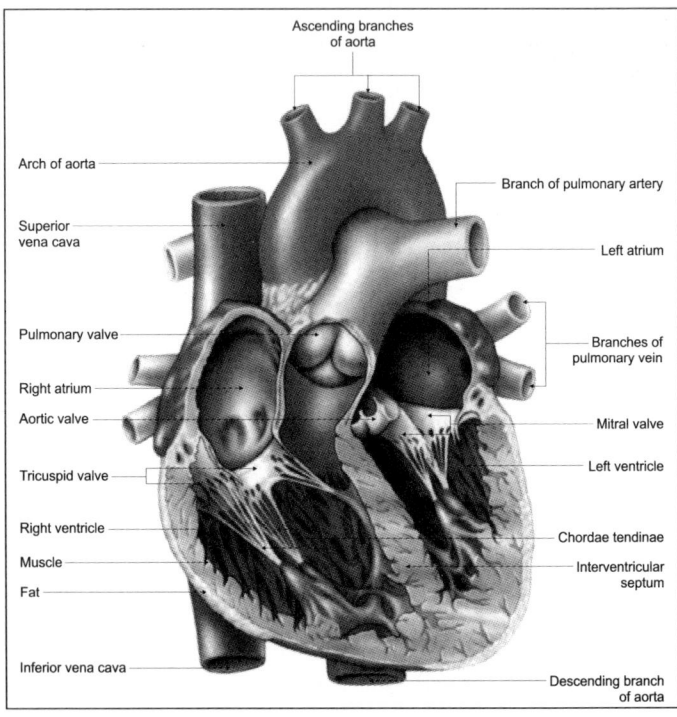

Fig. 4.9 View of the Heart

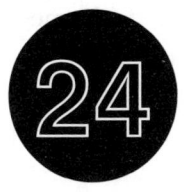

Peripheral Artery Disease

Peripheral Artery Disease (PAD) is caused by atherosclerotic narrowing of the arteries in the extremities. It is more like coronary artery disease and carotid artery disease where fatty deposits prevent proper flood flow through the arteries of the legs or arms. About 20 per cent of people over the age of sixty-five have peripheral artery disease.

The modifiable risk factors that can cause coronary heart disease can also cause atherosclerosis affecting the blood circulating in the peripheries. Claudication and chest pain are the main symptoms of PAD. Claudication is severe pain, more like cramps in the legs. Intermittent Claudication is where the pain comes and goes often with exercise and goes away with rest. In patients with severe limb, ischemia pain occurs even at rest. They may often feel tingling and prickling feelings in their fingers and toes.

Few tests that are used to diagnose peripheral vascular diseases are Ankle Brachial Pressure Index

(ABI), Doppler ultrasound, treadmill test, MRA and CT Angiogram. ABI is the ratio of blood pressures measured in the lower legs and arms. Lower blood pressure in the legs compared to the arm indicates peripheral artery disease. Patients with abnormal ABI have double the risk of having a heart attack, stroke or heart failure compared to people with normal ABI.

Patients with PAD frequently have associated coronary artery disease, carotid artery stenosis or cerebrovascular disease. About 28 per cent of people with PAD have a history of heart attack. Patients with PAD have upto a six-fold increase in risk of death due to cardiovascular disease.

People with peripheral artery disease need to modify their risk factors by quitting smoking or controlling hypertension. In addition, antiplatelet therapy to prevent clot formation and drugs to treat Claudication may be administered. Exercise rehabilitation can also help with symptoms.

Newer Risk Factors

Many patients who have a heart attack do have risk factors like high cholesterol or high blood pressure. More researches were done in the last few decades to evaluate new risk factors that caused atherosclerosis.

Some of the newer markers of inflammation are high sensitivity C-reactive protein (hsCRP), lipoprotein (a), homocysteine and fibrinogen.

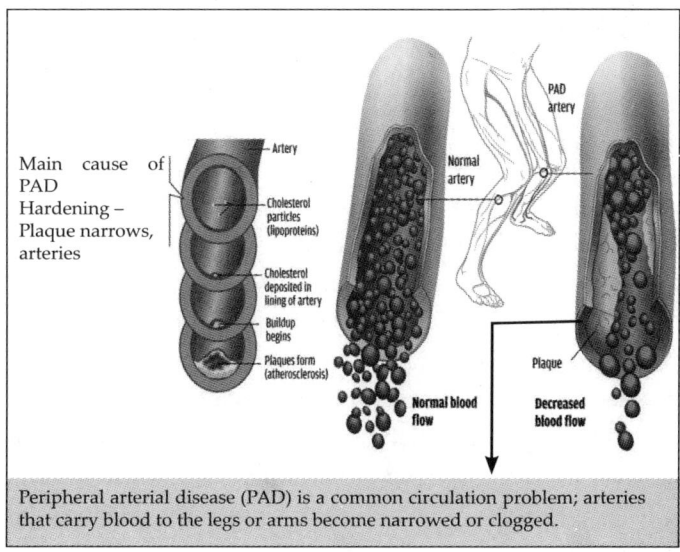

Fig. 4.10 Peripheral Artery Disease

Increased Homocysteine

Homocysteine is an amino acid which is synthesised in the body. High level of homocysteine in blood (homocysteinemia) is considered as a risk factor for early development of heart disease. Studies have shown increased levels of Homocysteine in people with familial premature coronary artery disease. Elevated Homocysteine levels are associated with vitamin B deficiency, especially folic acid, renal disease or hypothyroidism. Rarely homocysteinemia can be a hereditary condition. Homocystinuria is an inherited metabolic disorder which causes increased homocysteine accumulation in the serum and then excreted in the urine.

Homocysteinemia is thought to cause endothelial dysfunction, which leads to increase in platelet aggregation and oxidised LDL cholesterol. Endothelium is the layer of cells that line the lumen of the artery. Injury to the endothelium is the first step in atherosclerosis. More studies are underway to substantiate the relationship between Homocysteine and heart disease. Other conditions associated with homocysteinemia are stroke and blood clots in the other blood vessels including veins.

Blood tests to check Homocysteine level in blood may not be economical to everyone and there are no current recommendations for all heart patients to have this test done. Vitamin B, especially folate supplementation lowers the level of Homocysteine in blood.

High Sensitivity C Reactive Protein (hsCRP)

There are several blood tests that indicate the risk for coronary artery disease. One among them is high sensitivity C-reactive protein. CRP is a protein produced by the liver in response to an infection or inflammation. It is considered as an acute phase protein whose level increases in the blood during an arterial inflammation, may be due to coronary artery disease or peripheral artery disease. A positive C-reactive protein test signifies the presence of atherosclerosis. Very high levels of CRP are often found during a heart attack and may even be a marker for urgent revascularisation procedures such as angioplasty or bypass surgery.

American Heart Association classified CRP levels as given below

1.0 mg/L – Low risk

1.0 mg/L to 3.0 mg/L – Average risk

Above 3.0 mg/L – High risk

If CRP continues to be high after stabilising a heart attack patient, it indicates the presence of continued inflammation. This could mean instability during recovery and risk of another heart attack. The level of CRP in blood in stabilised patients may predict their outcome in the following year.

Your doctor might prescribe cholesterol lowering medications such as statins to reduce your CRP levels and risk for heart disease.

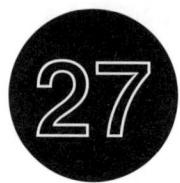

Lipoprotein (a)

Lipoprotein (a) or Lp (a) is a low density lipoprotein (LDL) particle with apoprotein A.

Lipoprotein (a) elevation can be inherited from parents. The apoprotein A has a structure similar to that of plasminogen, which can dissolve the blood clots around the atherosclerotic plaque. Apoprotein A attaches itself to the receptors of plasminogen and disturbs the anticlotting mechanism. Apoprotein A also causes more cells to accumulate around the plaque.

The average normal values of Lp (a) are 3.8mg/dl in men and 4.4mg/dl in women. The risk of heart disease increases three times when these levels of Lp (a) are above 30mg/dl. It causes coronary artery obstruction or re-obstruction resulting in a heart attack. High levels of lipoprotein (a) can cause atherosclerotic blockages in the arteries supplying the brain and legs.

It is important for people with elevated Lp (a) levels to keep other modifiable risk factors under control. Treatment to bring Lp (a) levels down are difficult. They cannot be lowered by diet or exercise, however healthy lifestyle can keep cholesterol and blood pressure levels normal. Daily use of Niacin may help lower lipoprotein (a) levels and increase HDL levels.

Fibrinogen

Fibrinogen is a protein that helps in blood clotting. It is a sticky coagulant that controls the blood's viscosity. With more fibrinogen the blood becomes more viscous. Since thicker blood flows less easily, there is a significant risk of increased fibrinogen causing heart attacks and strokes.

High levels of fibrinogen along with other risk factors such as smoking or hypertension elevated a person's chance of a hemorrhagic attack. Smoking and hypertension injures the artery walls and clotting agents are attracted to the injured site. Fibrinogen is one of the coagulants. Higher levels of fibrinogen promote thromboses (clot formation) and block the blood supply through the arteries.

Factors that are associated with high fibrinogen levels are smoking, overweight, high cholesterol levels, diabetes, high carbohydrate diet, stress, inactivity, oral contraceptives, genetics and old age. Fibrinogen rises and falls in blood in response to any stimuli such as stress or an infection.

High fibrinogen level is considered a symptom and a risk for coronary artery disease. Since fibrinogen increases in patients with heart disease and a person with high fibrinogen levels develop heart disease, it forms a vicious cycle. So it becomes essential to lower fibrinogen level. Factors that can lower fibrinogen in blood are exercise, no smoking and diets rich in vegetables and fish oil. Fibrates, a group of medications used to lower triglycerides, can be used to lower fibrinogen levels.

Severe Anaemia

Anaemia is a condition in which the haemoglobin content in the blood is below normal. Haemoglobin is a protein in the red blood cells which carries oxygen to the body parts. Anaemia can occur due to several causes such as iron deficiency, active bleeding, chronic kidney disease, poor nutrition and pregnancy.

Table 4.2 Severity of Anaemia based on Haemoglobin Values

Haemoglobin levels (g/dl)		Anaemia
Men 9.5 to 13	Women 9.5 to 11	Mild
8.0 to 9.5		Moderate
Less than 8.0		Severe

In patients with anaemia every tissue in the body receives less oxygen which leads to many symptoms. Fatigue, shortness of breath, malaise, dizziness and pallor are some of its symptoms. In patients with severe anaemia, the heart muscles do not get enough oxygen. The heart works harder, heart rate increases.

Continuous overload of the heart may lead to heart failure. Patients with chronic untreated anaemia have more chances of blocked atherosclerosis. Prolonged starvation of the heart muscles may even lead to a heart attack. Heart attacks even happen in anaemic adults with no prior history of coronary artery disease.

Most of the patients admitted with a heart attack have anaemia. It also increases the mortality rate in heart attack and heart failure patients. The prognosis worsens in patients with chronic diseases such as kidney insufficiency or diabetes.

Different types of anaemia may require different treatments. People may be treated with iron supplements or vitamins. Some may need medications to stimulate the production of red blood cells, while others require blood transfusion.

Infection

Studies now consider bacterial and viral infections could trigger or add on to the process of atherosclerosis. Though the evidence to support this concept is inadequate, bacteria named Chlamydia pneumoniae and certain viruses including cytomegalovirus (CMV) and herpes virus are considered as risk factors for heart disease. Infections in the artery and outside the vascular system could stimulate atherosclerosis. In patients with existing atherosclerosis, the balance in the clotting system may be lost when the body responds to an acute infection. This can cause an atherosclerotic plaque to rupture and cause a thrombus or emboli resulting in a heart attack.

Infections could aggravate heart disease by increasing the body temperature and heart rate. When this happens the body's metabolic demand is increased. This means more oxygen is supplied to the body while the heart is supplied with less than normal oxygen causing ischemia in heart patients.

Currently researchers are trying to prove if heart disease by infection is caused by direct damage on the artery wall or disturbances it causes in the body's metabolism and clotting system.

Chronic Kidney Disease

Renal insufficiency or renal failure is a condition when the kidneys no longer filter toxins and waste products from the blood properly. There is a decrease in the glomerular filtration rate or the rate at which fluid is filtered through the kidney. Diagnosis of kidney malfunction can be performed by a blood test called serum creatinine. In patients with renal insufficiency the serum creatinine level is elevated.

Most chronic kidney disease patients have other cardiovascular risk factors such as diabetes, hypertension or a history of smoking. Some more factors such as high levels of homocysteine, calcium and phosphorous in these patients also contribute to heart disease. Anaemia occurs and it often requires aggressive treatment in older people with renal insufficiency.

Chronic kidney disease patients are prone to have silent heart attacks along with arrhythmias and heart failure. Renal dysfunction is considered a highly inflammatory state which provides more chances for plaque ruptures in the coronary artery. Patients with renal disease have a high risk for heart disease and patients with end stage renal disease have high rates of mortality after a heart attack.

People with renal insufficiency are considered weak and have more side effects to medications. So unlike other people treated for a heart attack, they do not receive medications such as beta blockers, aspirin and thrombolytic therapy. Thrombolytic therapy may increase their risk of having a haemorrhage because of their abnormal platelet function. These patients are less likely to have angiogram or angioplasty. The contrast dye used during a catheterisation procedure increases serum creatinine levels and has adverse effect on the kidneys. The mortality rate after a heart attack in these patients may be high because of the medications or treatments they do not receive. Trials are being conducted to determine if drugs such as beta blockers will be more beneficial in patients with chronic kidney disease.

32 Idiopathic Pulmonary Fibrosis

Idiopathic pulmonary fibrosis or IPF is a progressive lung disease where the lung tissues become scarred. Mild scarring starts at the edges and progresses towards the lungs' centre. The cause of idiopathic pulmonary fibrosis is unknown. It can be inherited or caused due to air pollution.

Over the period of several months to years the normal tissues of the lungs are all replaced by scarred tissues. Breathing becomes very difficult and the oxygen supply to the body is compromised.

Symptoms of idiopathic pulmonary fibrosis are shortness of breath, dry cough, weight loss and fatigue. Complications such as lung failure, lung infections or cancer can occur. Patients with IPF are three times at risk for having a heart attack because the heart muscles constantly face oxygen starvation. These patients are also at increased risk for strokes and deep vein thrombosis.

While there are no medications currently to cure the disease, some drugs are used to slow down the process of scarring. Oxygen supplementation using a portable tank may be provided as palliative care. Some patients may be considered for lung transplant. Newer medications are currently being studied for treating this disease.

Systemic Lupus Erythematosus

Systemic Lupus Erythematosus (SLE) is a systemic autoimmune disease. An autoimmune disease is a disease where the body's immune system produces antibodies against its own cells. SLE is more common in women than in men. It can occur at any age. It harms several organs including skin, joints, heart, liver, lungs, nervous systems and kidneys. Arthritis, haemolytic anaemia, thrombocytopenia and pulmonary hypertension are some of the complications of this disease. It can also increase the risk of thrombosis in the arteries and veins. Immunosuppressants, and other medications are used to treat the symptoms. At present, there is no cure for this disease.

Systemic Lupus Erythematosus can even be drug-induced. There are hundreds of medications that can cause this disease; procainamide, hydralazine and quinidine, to name a few.

The heart problems associated with SLE are pericarditis, chest pain and pericardial tamponade.

Atherosclerosis can also occur or increase in patients with SLE. There can be rapid changes in the artery lumen in patients with existing coronary artery disease and a heart attack can occur even in young patients. There is an extremely high risk for middle-aged women with SLE to have a heart attack. Huge coronary artery aneurysm in patients with SLE usually causes an acute heart attack.

Patients with SLE should be treated aggressively for their coronary artery disease. Blood supply to the myocardium is also compromised, if there is thrombosis or an embolism due to endocarditis (inflammation of the heart's inner layers). Coronary arteritis or the inflammation of the coronary arteries can rarely occur with SLE. Abnormal heart rhythm can also occur as a complication.

Kawasaki Syndrome

Kawasaki Syndrome or Kawasaki disease is named after a Japanese doctor, Dr Tomisaku Kawasaki, who first described the disease in 1967. It is an autoimmune disease and one of the leading causes of acquired heart disease in children. It is also known as Mucocutaneous Lymph Node Syndrome. The cause of the disease is not known, but there are possibilities of genetic and environmental aspects. It occurs mostly in children under 5 years of age. Kawasaki disease was more prevalent in south Asian countries like Japan, Taiwan and Korea. It is now occurring more frequently in the United States and United Kingdom.

The disease causes high fever with eye infection, reddened and swollen mouth, lips and tongue. Other symptoms are swollen lymph glands, oedema in hands and feet with skin peeling and measles like rash.

Fever starts to subside in about a week or two. If the disease is left untreated, complications of the heart related complications occur. The most important complication is coronary artery aneurysm, which means the coronary artery walls start to expand. Thrombosis or rupture of the coronary artery can occur. When a blood clot occludes the coronary artery completely, it can result in a heart attack.

Any child presented with this syndrome should be admitted to the emergency department and treatment is directed towards slowing inflammation and preventing heart disease.

35

Familial Hypercholesterolemia

Familial Hypercholesterolemia is a genetic disorder which causes an increase in low-density lipoprotein (LDL) levels in blood. It affects about 1 in 500 people and usually, atleast one parent carries this gene. The occurrence of a child getting the gene from both parents is rare, but if that happens, the risk for heart disease is greatly amplified. In people with familial hypercholesterolemia, there is a high risk of developing coronary artery disease under the age of 40 in men and 50 in women.

The signs of familial hypercholesterolemia are:

- Xanthomas – Fatty skin deposits in lump forms in the tendons of the knees, elbows, feet, hand and the Achilles tendon
- Fat can deposit around the eyelids and in the cornea

The most common problem faced by people with this condition is atherosclerosis. Since atherosclerosis starts in a young age, the chances of a heart attack are very high. Family history of premature coronary artery disease also adds to the risk.

Family hypercholesterolemia can be diagnosed by a blood cholesterol test. Treatment will be aimed to reduce the LDL levels in the blood with the help of cholesterol lowering agents. Some may require very high doses or a combination of pills to lower the cholesterol levels.

 Fabry's Disease

Fabry's disease is a genetic, lysosomal storage disorder where an enzyme called alpha galactosidase becomes deficient. Glycolipids are carbohydrates and lipids attached together. These glycolipids accumulate abnormally in the tissues and blood vessels because of the enzyme deficiency.

Other names of Fabry's disease are:
- GLA deficiency or Alpha-galactosidase – A deficiency disease
- Anderson-Fabry disease
- Angiokeratoma coporis diffusum
- Ceramide Trihexosidase deficiency
- Hereditary dystopic lipidosis

Symptoms of this disease involve a range of organs. Kidney insufficiency or failure can occur. The corneas may appear clouded, although there is no vision damage. There can be other eye damages too including optic atrophy, conjunctival aneurysms and papilloedema. There can be papules appearing on the thighs, lower abdomen or groin area, which are usually painless. Tinnitus, neuropathy, fatigue and diarrhoea are also some of the symptoms of Fabry's disease.

When these glycolipids accumulate in the coronary artery walls, the risk for heart attack increases. Heart attack, stroke, abnormal heart rhythm and kidney failure are the common causes of death in people with Fabry's disease. This disease can thicken the walls of the ventricles and cause heart failure. It can also cause hypertension, which is also a known risk factor for heart attacks.

Enzyme replacement therapy to replace the deficient enzyme is one way of treating Fabry's disease and preventing potential complications. Pain medications and ACE inhibitors are also used in treating specific symptoms.

Hughes Syndrome

Hughes Syndrome is also known as antiphospholipid antibody syndrome and the sticky blood syndrome. People with this syndrome have an increased tendency to form blood clots in veins and arteries. This syndrome can occur alone or coexist with Systemic Lupus Erythematosus (SLE).

Hughes Syndrome is an auto-immune disorder which occurs more commonly in women than men. The cause of this disease is unknown. Several organs get affected because of antiphospholipid syndrome. Migraine, memory loss, deep vein thrombosis, stroke, visual disturbances and dizziness are some of its symptoms. Because of the blood clots, there is improper circulation of blood and the skin has a blotchy appearance. Ulcers can occur.

Women suffer severe pregnancy problems such as miscarriages, premature delivery or still birth. Clots in the heart can lead to heart attacks and upto 20 per cent of people under the age of 45, who suffered a heart attack, have this condition.

Treatment is generally aimed at thinning the blood and avoiding clot formations. Aspirin, clopidogrel, warfarin or heparin is used for anticoagulation.

Takayasu Arteritis

Takayasu Arteritis (TA) is a disease that causes chronic inflammation in large arteries, mainly the aorta and its major branches. It is a rare disease affecting more women than men in their second or third decade of life. The cause of this disease is unknown. This disease can cause narrowing of the arteries (stenosis) or abnormal dilation (aneurysms).

People with Takayasu's Arteritis often experience fatigue, claudication in the upper and lower extremities, night sweats, low grade fever, dizziness, chest pain and joint pain. High blood pressure, stroke and heart failure are some of the complications of Takayasu's Arteritis. The narrowing of arteries in this disease can also result in reduced blood flow to the heart muscles and cause a heart attack.

Treatment would aim at relieving inflammation of the arteries and preventing complications. When narrowing becomes severe, patients may require angioplasty or bypass surgery to re-establish blood flow through the arteries. Aneurysm repair surgery may be needed to prevent rupture of arteries.

39 Bland-White-Garland Syndrome

Bland-White-Garland Syndrome is also known as ALCAPA which stands for anomalous left coronary artery arising from the pulmonary artery. It is a rare congenital abnormality.

Normally, the coronary arteries arise from the aorta which carries oxygenated blood to the heart muscles. In this condition, the coronary artery receives blood from the pulmonary artery which carries deoxygenated blood. This condition is mostly diagnosed within the first two months of life.

Children are often fussy, irritable and have poor feeding habits. When the myocardium continues to receive oxygen-depleted blood, ischemia occurs. Increase in myocardial demand can lead to a heart attack. Heart failure, chest pain and sudden death occur in some.

Supportive medical treatment is given to provide relief from symptoms and surgery is necessary to correct the anomaly.

Polyarteritis Nodosa

Polyarteritis Nodosa is a disease that causes inflammation of medium sised arteries and impairs the flow of blood through them. The cause of this disease is unknown, although about 20 per cent of people with polyarteritis nodosa have Hepatitis-B. It is a rare disorder that can occur at any age, but more between the ages of 40 and 60. Men and women are equally prone to this disease.

Symptoms are usually related to the organs that are affected; some of the general symptoms are fatigue, fever, joint pain, decreased appetite, weight loss and abdominal pain. About 50 per cent of these patients have musculoskeletal symptoms. Inflammatory changes of the skin including painful nodules and ulcers can occur. The ulcers with more loss of blood supply can become gangrene. If the arteries in the central nervous system are inflamed, it can lead to epilepsy or stroke. Kidney failure can occur. Cardiac symptoms occur in about ten to 30 per cent of the patients. When the coronary arteries are involved, heart attack and heart failure can occur.

Immunosuppressants and steroids are used to improve symptoms in patients with polyarteritis nodosa. In people with Hepatitis infection, antiviral medications are also essential. Other treatments may depend on the organs that are involved.

Rheumatoid Vasculitis

Rheumatoid Vasculitis is a rare but very serious complication of rheumatoid arthritis. It can occur in both men and women at any age. Usually, these patients have long standing rheumatoid arthritis with many joint involvements and the concentration of rheumatoid factor in their blood is high. Vasculitis means inflammation of the blood vessels. The inflammation weakens, thickens, narrows or dilates the blood vessels.

Rheumatoid vasculitis involves the blood vessels of skin, nervous system, the sclera of the eye, fingers and toes. The amount of damage caused depends on the size of the arteries or veins that are involved. The involvement of larger arteries in rheumatoid vasculitis is rare. When involved, they can cause occlusion and completely cut blood supply to that particular organ. In addition to stroke and gangrene of the fingers and toes, heart attacks can occur when the blood supply to the myocardium is cut off.

Treatment of rheumatoid vasculitis depends on the size of the vessels and the organs involved. Cortisone drugs, such as prednisone, are used to control the inflammation and suppress the immune system. More medications may be needed to treat skin ulcers or other internal organ damages.

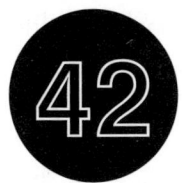

Cocaine

Cocaine, because of its prevalent use, is a well-known cause of heart attack and sudden cardiac death. Studies over the past forty years have shown that cocaine abuse was the reason for sudden death in young adults.

Even small amounts of cocaine ingestion can cause constriction of the coronary arteries decreasing oxygen supply to the myocardium. It can also increase myocardial oxygen demand in heart patients by accelerating atherosclerosis, platelet aggregation and clot formation. Cocaine users with coronary artery disease have a very high risk of myocardial ischemia and heart attack.

Cocaine is known to cause endothelial structural abnormality, thereby increasing the amount of LDL or bad cholesterol to enter the arteries. It also increases the concentration of plasminogen activator inhibitor to increase clot accumulation.

The most common heart related symptom associated with cocaine users is chest pain. People who get cardiac symptoms may not always be habitual cocaine users. Even first time users or recreational users can injure the heart muscles often within minutes of cocaine use. Most of them are young male smokers. The effects of smoking along with cocaine are detrimental.

Complications after a heart attack induced by cocaine such as arrhythmias, heart failure or death are uncommon. As the concentration of the drug declines in the body, the blood vessels begin to relax again and resupplying blood to the myocardium.

Amphetamine

Amphetamine is a drug that comes under the class of phenethylamine. It is a psycho-stimulant that was once used for the treatment of attention deficit disorder, narcolepsy and obesity. Nowadays their use is strictly limited. Inspite of it being illegal to use without a prescription some people use it as performance enhancers or recreational drugs. Few of the commonly abused amphetamines are dextroamphetamine, methcathinone, methylphenidate, ephedrine, phenmetrazine and MMDA also known as ecstasy.

Meth or crystal meth or ICE is another form of amphetamines that look like ice crystals and it can be smoked, injected or snorted. Along with extensive heart damage, crystal meth can be harmful to the liver, kidneys and brain. Users of methamphetamine have five fold risks of strokes and heart attacks. It is very addictive since it can cause powerful highs very quickly. An overdose of crystal meth can cause coma or cardiac arrest.

The effects of amphetamines on the heart are similar to cocaine use. Amphetamines may cause spasm of the coronary arteries with or without clot formation. It also increases the heart's workload by increasing heart rate and blood pressure. Even young adults under amphetamine abuse can suffer fatal heart attacks.

People who are addicted to amphetamines have less appetite, increased nervousness, tremors and sensitivity to noise. Apart from having heart problems amphetamine users face memory loss, psychological problems and even dental issues.

Oxycodone

Oxycodone is an analgesic medication used to treat moderate to severe pain. It belongs to a class of drugs called opiate. It changes the way the central nervous system responds to pain. It is commonly found in combinations with acetaminophen or ibuprofen.

Oxycodone is available in the form of capsules, tablets, concentrated solution and extended release tablets. It should be taken only as directed by the physician. Oxycodone is started at a low dose initially and if pain is uncontrolled over time the dose may be increased. If you are taking this for a long time, it should not be stopped suddenly. There may be several symptoms when you withdraw this medicine you may have symptoms such as watery eyes, sneezing, yawning, chills, joint aches, muscle pains, irritability, anxiety, cramps, diarrhoea, vomiting, depression and fast heart rate.

There are several side effects which include memory loss, nausea, constipation, dizziness, memory loss, anxiety, euphoria and increased sweating. In higher doses it can be lethal. It slows down the heart rate, shallow breathing and decreases the heart rate and make can breathing shallow. It can lead to a sudden arrest in breathing, cardiac arrest, coma or death.

People who have been addicted to oxycodone or other narcotics are at an increased risk for hepatitis, skin infections, tetanus, strokes or heart attacks. It is essential that they seek help immediately. They may need counseling and medical help to recover completely.

 # Air Pollution

Nowadays, everybody is exposed to some degree of air pollution. Short term or long term effects of the pollution depends on the amount of pollutants that you are exposed to. Researches done in the last decade has shown that a consistent exposure to large amount of pollutants is a huge risk factor for cardiovascular disease and stroke. People with existing heart or lung disease, elderly ad diabetics are at increased risk.

Some of the components that pollute the air are carbon monoxide, smokes from cigarettes or cigars, nitrates, sulfur dioxide and particulate matter. Particulate matters are solid or liquid particles generated from automobile emission, industries, metal processing, smelting, generating power, burning wood, pollen, forest fires, volcano, dust from road and mold. These tiny particles when inhaled are capable of killing thousands of people every year.

Nitrogen dioxide is found indoors from the use of gas stoves and kerosene heaters. High traffic areas, power plant emissions and fossil burning can also be sources of nitrogen dioxide.

Cigarette smoking, including secondhand smokes contribute to indoor pollution and affects the heart and the vascular system. Inhaling smokes from just one cigarette a day can increase the progress of coronary artery disease. Carbon monoxide is present in cigarette smokes and vehicle combustion. They also decrease the amount of oxygen carried to the body and heart.

Studies have shown that when diesel exhausts are inhaled in high concentration, normal blood clotting activity is disrupted. Long term exposure to air pollution hardens arteries. These harmful effects raise the chances of having a heart attack. When large amounts of particulate matter are inhaled, it decreases the life expectancy by a few yeas.

Carbon Monoxide Poisoning

Carbon monoxide is an invisible tasteless and odourless gas. It can be detected only by installing carbon monoxide detectors. It can be present in your home or work. Initially it causes symptoms such as nausea, vomiting and headaches. Dizziness, shortness of breath an even coma can occur when there is moderate exposure to carbon monoxide. When exposed to higher levels, the outcome is dangerous and deadly. It can result in severe brain damage or a heart attack due to hypoxia. It is the most common cause of accidental poisoning and is called the invisible killer.

Household appliances are the most common source of carbon monoxide. Gas water heaters, smokes from fires, kerosene heaters, charcoal grills, car exhausts, cigarette smokes, paint removers, degreasers, solvents and paints are some of the sources of carbon monoxide.

When high amounts of carbon monoxide are present in the blood, the body's ability to deliver oxygen to the internal organs is reduced. Moreover carbon monoxide directly affects the heart muscles and reduces its capability to pump efficiently. Carbon monoxide poisoning has a long standing effect on the myocardium and it is critical to prevent it. Children, foetuses, elderly and people with heart or lung disease are more susceptible to carbon monoxide poisoning. There is an increased risk of mortality in people with heart attacks due to carbon monoxide poisoning.

When you suspect carbon monoxide poisoning it is necessary to get to an emergency department immediately. Also it is possible that more than one family member is affected at the same time. High dose oxygen supply is given to treat this poisoning. Also it is necessary to repair the source of high carbon monoxide levels in your home or work.

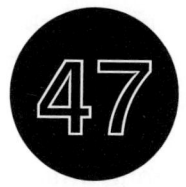

Mediastinal Irradiation

Thoracic irradiation to treat breast cancer or Hodgkin's lymphoma has some damaging effects on the heart. The irradiation causes inflammation and fibrosis of the heart's structures including its layers, muscles, valves and arteries. Many of the cancer survivors who received radiation years ago are now being treated for cardiovascular diseases.

About 30 per cent of the patients who received mediastinal irradiation had cardiac complications. Most patients developed symptoms like chest pain during the course of radiation therapy. The most common cardiac complication is pericarditis or inflammation of the outer layer of the heart. Along with valve dysfunction, cardiomyopathy and fibrosis of the heart's muscle, coronary artery disease seemed to be prevalent. A majority of cardiac related deaths in these patients are due to a heart attack.

The risk of a heart attack is increased with certain chemotherapy medications which are used along with radiation. Other known cardiac risk factors such as tobacco, high cholesterol or hypertension increase the chances of coronary artery disease and heart attack. Most patients who received radiation and died suddenly of a heart attack did not have the conventional risk factors. These risk factors when present must be treated aggressively to inhibit heart disease progression.

Periodical evaluation for heart disease is useful when people are treated to moderately high doses of irradiation. When patients with coronary artery disease are identified, procedures such as angioplasty or bypass surgery may improve their outcomes.

When newer strategies such as lower does of radiation, not using cardio-toxic chemotherapy agents and minimal exposure of the heart are employed the risk of heart disease is reduced.

Severe Anaphylactic Reaction

Anaphylaxis, a word derived from Greek, means 'against protection'. Anaphylactic reaction is an allergic reaction that may be severe and life-threatening. The whole body is usually affected and, at times, under a few minutes.

Anaphylactic reactions can be caused due to bee stings, food allergies including peanuts, drug allergy, insect venom, latex or even, pollen allergies. Usually the person is exposed to the substance in the past and develops a reaction that sometimes even goes unnoticed or has no reaction at all. This is termed as sensitisation.

Some of the symptoms of an anaphylactic reaction are:

1. Itching
2. Hives/Rashes
3. Breathing problems and/or Wheezing
4. Coughing
5. Dizziness
6. Loss of consciousness
7. Fast Heart rate
8. Anxiety
9. Confusion
10. Cardiac arrest

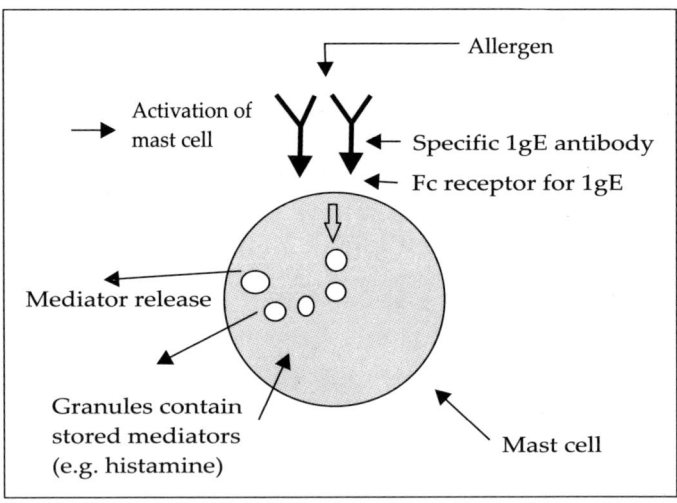

Fig. 4.11

Studies have shown that 'anaphylaxis-induced myocardial ischemia' or a heart attack induced by anaphylaxis is caused by several mechanisms and in variable combinations. Histamine is released from mast cells in large quantities during an anaphylactic reaction. This can cause coronary vasospasm even in people with normal coronary arteries. In people with existing coronary artery disease, histamine can destabilise the plaque and may even rupture it.

Another mechanism is that anaphylaxis can cause a sudden drop in blood pressure for a long period, causing reduced blood flow to the heart muscles. Existing blockage in the coronary arteries along with prolonged hypotension can result in heart attacks.

Severe Burns

Skin exposed to heat from fire, chemicals, radiation, electricity or hot liquids can cause a burn. Even too much exposure to the sun can cause burns. Based on the amount of skin affected burns may be classified as first, second or third degree burns. First degree burn is when only the outer layer of the skin is affected and second degree burn is extended to the dermis or the layer underneath the skin. Third degree burns involves not just the skin, but also muscles, tendons and bones.

The most common complications of burns are infection and dehydration. Depending on the extent and severity, emergency medical attention is necessary. First degree burns can be treated at home. Running cool water on the burnt area for several minutes decreases further heat from spreading. Butter, Vaseline or oil should not be applied to the burn wounds. Ice cubes should not be placed directly on the wound but a cold compress may be used. Ibuprofen or acetaminophen reduces pain.

A third degree burn can cause the heart rate and blood pressure to increase. Unless intravenous fluid is given to resuscitate the fluid loss, the heart will not be able to meet the body's state of increased metabolism. Fluid volume shifts in the tissues and there is relatively less blood flowing in the body. The amount of blood pumped out by the heart (cardiac output) also decreases. This will lead to reduced oxygen supply to the heart muscles and a heart attack can occur as a complication. People who suffer burns from fire injury may sustain carbon monoxide poisoning. This also causes the coronary arteries to constrict and restrict the amount of blood flowing through it.

Third degree burns require immediate treatment and hospitalisation. Healing may include scarring in some people with third degree burns. If ninety per cent of the body surface is burnt the results are often fatal.

Pain killers, antibiotics, IV fluids, skin care and proper diet can be part of treatment options. Some patients may require skin grafting surgery, physical and occupational therapy. Some may face depression when disfiguring or scarring occurs. Medications or psychotherapy is required to relieve depression.

Sepsis causing hypotension

Sepsis can be also termed as blood poisoning. It is a life threatening condition that occurs due to infections in the body. The organisms enter the bloodstream and cause the whole body to produce an inflammatory response. Severe sepsis causes abnormal functioning of the organs.

Patients with sepsis have elevated heart rate and respiratory rate. Their body temperature could be either above or below normal. The white blood cells in the blood that fight against infections are abnormally high. Sepsis rapidly progresses and causes a state of shock where the blood pressure falls and mental status is altered. There is more clot formation in the blood.

Severe hypotension can lead to less oxygen supply to the muscles. Angina or heart attack occur secondary to coexisting coronary artery disease in septic patients. Several factors that depress the myocardium such as cytokines, prostanoids and nitric oxide are found in the blood during sepsis. Myocardial dysfunction starts within hours after the onset of sepsis and involves both the ventricles.

Adequate and prompt antibiotic therapy along with intravenous fluids and medications to maintain blood pressure are given to treat sepsis. Oxygen may be supplemented in patients with decreased oxygen saturation.

Chapter 5

Tests to Diagnose Coronary Artery Disease

Chest pain, shortness of breath and palpitations are few of the symptoms that trigger suspicion of heart disease. Your physician would question you further about your symptoms and get a complete medical history including your family history and social history. Social history would include smoking, alcohol habits, lifestyle and job related factors.

He would then do a physical examination. This would include measuring your heart rate, blood pressure and listen to your hearts and lungs with a stethoscope. He may even check for pulses in your neck, legs and feet. This is done to rule out carotid artery disease and peripheral artery diseases.

Finally to diagnose coronary artery disease, he may put you through a series of diagnostic tests.

Nowadays, people though asymptomatic may have these tests done during their annual physicals or for health insurance purposes.

The tests that are normally associated with the heart are:

1. Electrocardiogram
2. Echocardiogram
3. Chest X ray
4. Stress test
a. Pharmacological Stress test
b. Nuclear stress test
c. Stress Echocardiogram
5. Cardiac catheterisation and angiogram

Newer methods to look at the coronary arteries are:

1. Computer Tomography (CT) Angiogram
2. Magnetic Resonance Angiogram (MRA)

Electrocardiogram (ECG or EKG)

An electrocardiogram is a recording of the heart's electrical activity. It is usually displayed and stored in a monitor and the tracings are printed onto a graph sheet.

The electrocardiogram is one of the oldest, simplest and indispensable methods of diagnosing several heart problems. It can tell us the heart rate, heart rhythm, presence of certain congenital heart diseases, structural abnormalities, less blood supply to the heart and even detect a heart attack.

What should you expect during an electrocardiogram?

It is a non invasive procedure. There is no pain involved. You will be asked to lie down on your back and unbutton your shirt. Several electrode patches will be placed on your chest, hands and feet. The conductive gel in the patches may feel cold. Leads from the ECG machine will be connected to the electrodes and a graph will be obtained in the monitor. The test takes less than a minute. There is no need to fast. Your doctor can review the results during the same visit.

Echocardiography (Echo)

An echocardiography is an ultrasound of the heart. An ultrasound uses sound waves to be sent into your body which are reflected back by your body's internal structures. The reflected sound is also referred as echo. A microphone like device called transducer sends and receives these sound waves. An echocardiography can help us see the heart's size and structures on a monitor. It can help diagnose structural abnormalities, abnormal flow patterns inside the heart, myocardial damage and valve problems. Even the pumping efficiency of the heart can be calculated.

What should you expect during an echocardiogram?

Echocardiogram is also a non invasive procedure. You may be asked to remove your shirt and wear the hospital gown. You will lie down on your back and may be asked to shift to your side. You will be requested to stay still. ECG electrodes may be placed on you so that they can get a simultaneous recording of electrocardiogram. The test is painless but the technician may push the transducer slightly on your chest. There will be lubricating gel on the transducer which may feel cold. Depending on what the doctor is looking for, this test takes about 30 minutes to one hour. There is no need to fast. Your doctor may send you home and call you with results later or discuss the results during the same visit. Sometimes a different cardiologist may read the echocardiogram and provide the report to your doctor.

Chest X-Ray

A chest X-ray is simply an X-ray of your chest. It can provide valuable information about lungs, heart, ribs, diaphragm and other structures in your chest. It can tell us the size and shape of the heart and show presence of calcium deposits in coronary arteries or heart valves. It also provides information on the lung condition. Lung tumour, pneumonia and many other medical problems can be diagnosed using a chest X-ray.

What should you expect during a chest X-ray?

Chest X-ray is a painless non-invasive procedure. You will be asked to remove all metal jewellery before having an X-ray. You will be requested to remove your shirt and wear a hospital gown. You will be asked to

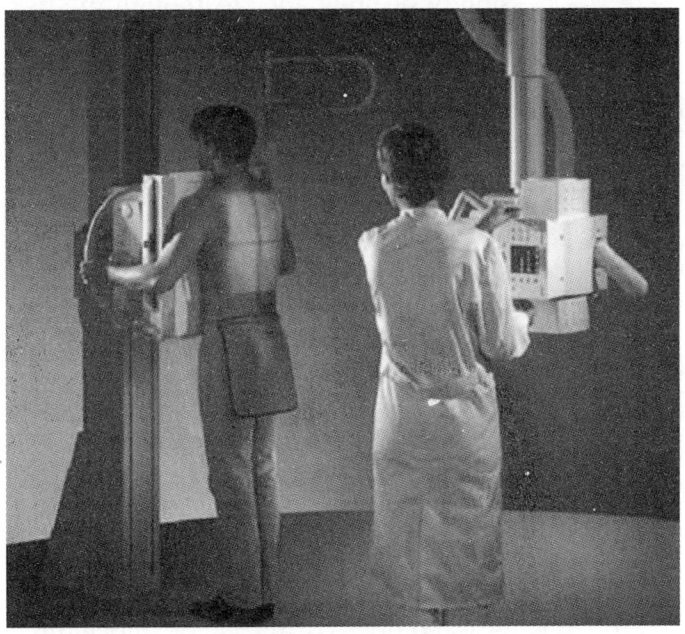

Fig. 5.1 Chest X-ray

stand against a plate containing the X-ray film. For the later view, you will be asked to stand with your side against the plate with the corresponding arm raised. The technologist will ask you to hold the breath while the picture is being taken. The test takes only less than 15 minutes.

There is a negligible amount of radiation involved in any X-ray procedures, but there is no harm from it. Women should inform their doctor or technician if there is a possibility of pregnancy. Although the risk of harming the unknown child is very less, doctors will take special precautions to prevent the baby's exposure.

Stress Test

A stress test is performed to see how your heart responds to exertion. This test is also called as treadmill test or stress electrocardiogram. Underlying ischemic heart disease may not be recorded during a normal electrocardiogram. But when a person exerts himself the oxygen supply to his myocardium can be reduced. There is a 70 per cent change of confirming coronary artery disease with a stress test. A stress test can also detect abnormal heart rhythms that are triggered during exercise.

What should you expect during a stress test?

You may be asked not to drink, eat or smoke three hours or more prior to a stress test. You will be asked to take your prescription medications as usual, unless the doctor orders you otherwise. Give the doctor a list of all your current medications.

Like an electrocardiogram, there will be patches stuck on to your chest, arm and legs. Wires from these patches will be connected to the ECG machine. It is better to wear comfortable clothes and a running shoe. You will be also connected to a blood pressure cuff and the technician will check your blood pressure periodically during the test.

Usually the test involves you to walk on a treadmill or pedal a stationary exercise bicycle. The speed and inclination of the treadmill or resistance on the bicycle will increase as the test progresses. The test will normally start when you reach your target heart rate when no symptoms occur.

At anytime during the test if you feel you are unable to continue, you must notify the technician immediately. Chest pain, shortness of breath or dizziness may occur if there is an underlying medical problem. The technician may stop the test if there are any major rhythm problems in the ECG or your blood pressure becomes too high or low.

The actual test may take only 15 minutes or less, but the preparation time may take 15 minutes more. Once the test is complete, you will be asked to lie down until your vital signs are back to normal.

Pharmacological Stress Test

A pharmacological stress test is advised when patients have limitations such as back trouble and arthritis that prevent them from walking on a treadmill. This test involves injecting medications such as dobutamine or adenosine to increase your heart rate instead of physical exercise. You will have an intravenous (IV) line, which will be removed after the test is complete. Like a regular stress test, ECG will be taken and blood pressure will be monitored.

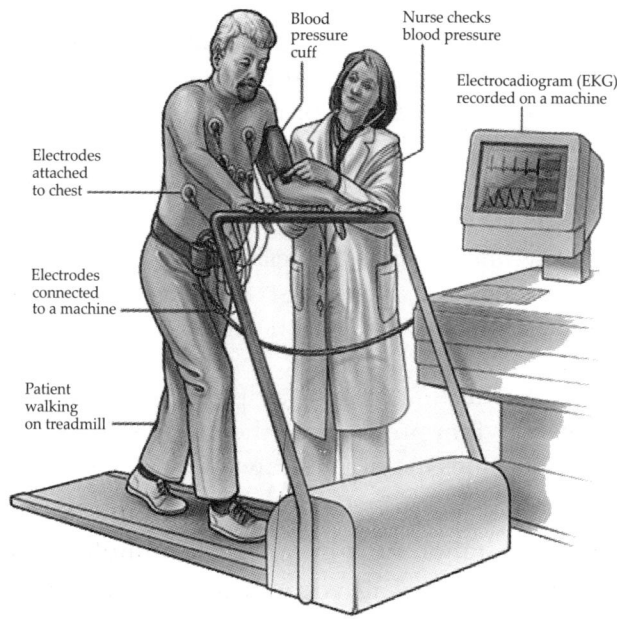

Fig 5.2 Pharmacological Stress Test

Nuclear Stress Test

This type of stress test involves injecting a small amount or radioactive material into the patient's vein. Thallium or Cardiolite are the commonly used isotopes. Nuclear images of the heart will be obtained prior to and immediately after exercising. When the two images are compared, any areas of the heart muscle will less blood supply will be visible. This type of testing is expensive when compared to a regular stress test and requires more time, but it is more accurate in diagnosing coronary artery disease. Usually, the imaging part takes about 20-30 minutes, when you will be asked to remain still.

Stress Echocardiogram

An exercise stress echocardiogram is an echocardiogram done along with exercise. This test can tell us how well your heart works under stress. Usually, the test begins with taking the pictures of your heart by an echo when you are resting. A resting electrocardiogram also will be done. Then you will be asked to exercise on a treadmill or your heart rate will be increased with medicines. Once your target heart rate is achieved, another echocardiogram will be done immediately. Some of the heart muscles may not receive enough blood supply during exercise. These areas can be visualised during a stress echocardiogram. The whole procedure may take upto 60 minutes including preparation time.

Cardiac Catheterisation and Angiogram

Cardiac catheterisation is an invasive procedure where a long, thin, flexible tube called a catheter is inserted into a blood vessel and sent to your heart. Cardiac catheterisation can be done to measure blood pressure inside the arteries and heart chambers. The catheter can contain a device at its tip to measure oxygen level in blood. It can be used to obtain tissues for biopsy. A balloon catheter can be used to treat coronary artery disease or valve diseases.

An angiogram is a type of cardiac catheterisation where dye or liquid contrast agents are injected into the coronary artery via the catheter. X-ray motion pictures are taken as the agent fills the arteries and any narrowing of the coronary artery lumen because of atherosclerosis can be seen. An angiography can accurately tell the per centage of blockage in each coronary artery and can be considered as the final test of diagnosis. Left ventriculography is commonly done along with coronary angiogram which detects the left ventricle's pumping efficiency.

What should you expect during an angiogram?

An elective angiogram will require you to be hospitalised the night before the procedure. You should not eat or drink atleast 8 hours before the procedure. You may be allowed to have small sips of water. Discuss with your doctor if you can take all your medications as usual.

You will be asked to change into a hospital gown. An intravenous line will be placed. A sedative will be given to ease anxiety. The area where the catheter will be inserted is usually the groin or an arm is cleaned well and local anaesthesia will be given to numb the site. You will be awake during the whole procedure but should not feel any pain or discomfort. The procedure will take only upto 30 minutes, but you will be kept in a recovery room. There will be pressure bandage on the place where the catheter was inserted. You will be asked to remain lying down to prevent strain on the puncture site.

You will be told to drink lots of water to remove the contrast agent from your body. Depending on your recovery, you may be allowed to start walking within 8 hours after the procedure and may be even sent home the same day or the very next day.

Computed Tomography (CT) Angiogram

A Computed tomography angiogram is an imagine technique to view your coronary arteries using X-ray. Part of the X-ray machine rotates rapidly around your body and takes images from all angles. Unlike a regular angiogram it does not involve a catheter being inserted into your artery. The dye to visualize the coronary artery will be injected through an intravenous line. The positive aspects of a CT angiogram are that it can diagnose coronary artery disease at an early stage and it is non-invasive. Location and size of calcium deposits in the arteries can be also found. A CT angiogram can be also used to assess diseases of the aorta and carotid artery stenosis.

Since a CT angiogram involves X-ray, you will be exposed to some amount of radiation. Tell your doctor if you are pregnant. Although the recovery time is less compared to a traditional coronary angiogram, the latter has an option of treating coronary artery disease by angioplasty at the time of the test itself.

What should you expect during a computed tomography angiogram?

A CT angiogram is done in a hospital or in an outpatient setting. You will be asked not to eat or drink for several hours before the test, especially if a contrast dye is going to be used. You may be allowed to drink water but caffeinated beverages should be avoided as it can increase your heart rate. Your doctor might ask you some medications before the test.

You may be requested to remove clothes waist up and change into a hospital gown. All metal objects including jewellery, hairpins, eye glasses, dentures, etc needs to be removed. An intravenous (IV) line will be inserted to inject the dye. You will lie on a long narrow table that slides through a small tunnel shaped machine that contains the X-ray tube and detectors. During the procedure you will be alone in the exam room. The technician will be in the computer room operating the machine that is separated by a glass window. He will be able to see, talk and hear you at all times. You will be asked to stay still during the test and may be asked to hold your breath for a few seconds. The actual test may take less than 15 minutes, but the preparation time might be longer. You should be able to continue with your normal activities after the test is complete.

Magnetic Resonance Angiogram (MRA)

Magnetic Resonance Angiogram (MRA) is a procedure that uses powerful magnetic field and radiofrequency waves to get cross sectional images of the body. With the help of a computer, these images are reconstructed to form 3-dimensional images. The MRA machine has a narrow table that slides through a cylindrical magnet. MRA can help diagnose several cardiovascular problems along with evaluating coronary artery disease. MRA can be done with or without the use of contrast dye. When the dye is used, it will be injected intravenously in an arm. MRA is also used in individuals after a stroke or diagnose blood vessel problems such as aneurysms.

142 | 50 Things That Cause Heart Attack

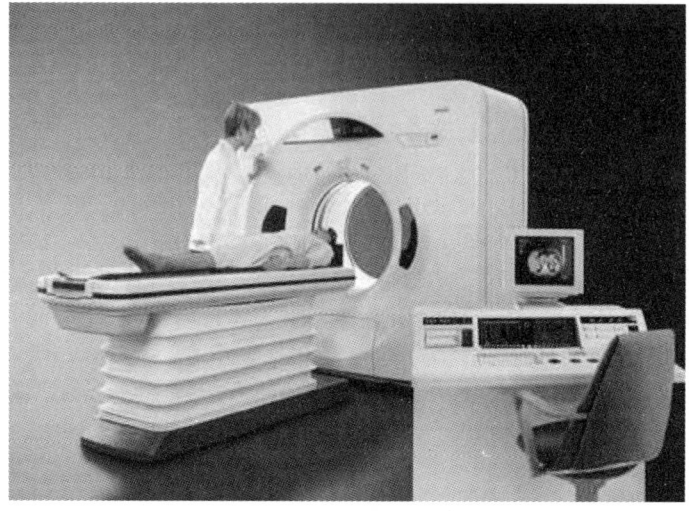

Fig. 5.3 MRA

What should you expect during a MRA?

You may be asked to change into a hospital gown. All metal objects such as jewelry, pen, hair pins and dentures must be left outside the scan room. If you have a pacemaker, surgical clips or any other metal implant, you must inform your doctor earlier. Inform your doctor if you are pregnant. People who are claustrophobic can request a sedative to relieve anxiety. You may be asked not to eat or drink anything few hours prior to the examination. An intravenous line may be placed if contrast dye is being used. You will be asked to lie still on the table and even hold your breath for a few seconds. There may be straps on you to help you maintain the proper position for imaging. You may be offered ear plugs or head phones as the MRA machine can produce loud clanging noises. The technician will be in a separate glass room but will be able to communicate with you at all times. The whole test including preparation may take up to an hour. After the test you may resume your normal activities.

Since these tests are relatively new, a cardiologist may consider a traditional angiogram to be the gold standard test to confirm coronary artery disease. These tests may not be widely used since the equipment is expensive and some hospitals may not have it.

Chapter 6
Treatment Options

Medical

The treatment for coronary artery disease and its duration depends upon the risk factors, symptoms and the severity of the disease. Doctors aim at reducing the associated symptoms and slowing the progression of the disease. They prescribe medication to decrease your chances of having a heart attack. Medications will be the first line of treatment in patients whose symptoms are minimal and the blood flow through the coronary artery is not severely restricted.

The knowledge medical professionals have gained over the past few years has helped them to keep an ailing heart pumping effectively. In addition to preventing a heart attack, medicines are given to decrease the chances of arrhythmias and heart failure. These advances have taken decades to reach us, but on the brighter side, there is an increase in life expectancy of the people suffering from coronary artery disease.

It is wise to carry a list containing the name of your medicines and dosage at all times. This list should include all non-prescription medicines such as multivitamins or any herbal supplements you take regularly. It would help a doctor prevent potential drug interactions. This list can provide lifesaving information to emergency medical professionals. All medications have generic and different brand names. Write down the generic name next to the brand name. The list should also contain the names of medications you are allergic to.

Before starting a medication, here are a few questions you must discuss with your doctor.

1. Why am I taking this pill? How should I take it?
2. What are its potential side effects? Are there any long term effects? Can I take over the counter pills to treat side effects like headaches or stomach upsets?
3. What should I do if I miss a dose? Can I take one as soon as I remember or should I wait for the next dose?
4. Will these pills affect my day-to-day activities in any way?

5. Are there any foods that I should refrain from in order to avoid drug interaction?
6. Will there be any blood tests done later because I'm taking this pill?
7. Is this pill potentially risky to a pregnant or a nursing woman?

Aspirin

Aspirin, also known as acetylsalicylic acid or ASA, has several uses. Most often, people use it to treat fevers or minor aches and pains. Physicians advise people with a history of heart attack or angina to take an aspirin everyday to prevent a heart attack. For people with coronary artery disease, aspirin acts as an anti-platelet, preventing platelets to aggregate in the blood vessel and form blood clots. Unless there are known allergies, everybody is given aspirin during a heart attack to reduce the impact and avoid heart muscles from dying. Long-term aspirin is also used to help prevent strokes. Stomach ulcers and risk of bleeding are some of the known side-effects of using long-term aspirin. To minimise these side-effects, regular aspirin can be replaced by baby aspirin.

Clopidogrel

Clopidogrel is commonly known by its brand name Plavix. It is an anti-platelet that prevents platelets to aggregate in arteries and form harmful blood clots that causes a heart attack. People who have undergone an angioplasty, especially with stent placements, are prescribed clopidogrel. There is a risk of increased bleeding with clopidogrel, so would be asked to stop taking it days before elective surgery. Discuss with your doctor if you are pregnant, have stomach ulcers or had a recent injury. Few other side-effects of clopidogrel are headache, dizziness, stomach pain, nose bleed and excessive tiredness.

Beta Blockers

Beta blockers, also known as beta-adrenergic blockers, are agents that reduce heart rate and blood pressure. They can make the heart pump efficiently with less force. Hence, it is an important medication in treating heart failure. When the supply of oxygen is reduced to the heart muscles, you develop chest pain. Beta blockers reduce the myocardium's need of oxygen thereby reducing the severity of angina. Studies have shown that beta blockers reduce the risk of early death during a heart attack. It is also used to treat certain abnormal heart rhythms. Generic names of a few beta blocking agents are Propranolol, Metoprolol, Labetalol, Carvedilol, Atenolol, Bisoprolol and Nadolol.

Fatigue, depression and abnormal slowing of heart beat are some of the side effects of beta blockers. Beta blockers have to be used with caution for people with diabetes, asthma, bronchitis or emphysema.

Calcium Channel Blockers

Cardiac muscles or myocardium require calcium ions to contract. Calcium channel blockers restrict the entry of calcium ions into the myocardium, thus lowering the force with which the muscles contract. So, the demand of oxygen supply by the myocardium is reduced, which in turn prevents angina attacks. Calcium channel blockers also lower blood pressure and treat certain abnormal heart rhythms. Generic names of a few calcium channel-blocking agents are Diltiazem, Verapamil, Amlodepine, Nifedipine, Nicardipine and Felodipine.

Some of the side effects associated with calcium channel blockers are very low blood pressure, leg oedema, slow heart rate and headache.

Ace-Inhibitors

ACE stands for Angiotensin converting enzyme. This medication was primarily developed to treat hypertension. ACE-inhibitors are prescribed to patients after a heart attack and with some decrease in their left ventricular function. When the blood pressure is reduced by ACE-inhbitors, the heart does not face much resistance in pumping blood out through the arteries. This can prevent a heart failure. ACE-inhibitors are also known to reduce the chance of a second heart attack. Generic names of a few ACE-inhibitors are Captopril, Enalapril, Ramipril, Lisinopril, Fosinopril and Quinapril. Side effects associated with Ace-inhibitors are chronic cough, flushing, dizziness and headache.

Diuretics

Diuretics, commonly known as the 'water pill', promote the kidneys to remove more water from the body. People with heart failure tend to accumulate water in their feet, ankles or abdomen. Diuretics are given to decrease this oedema. It is also known to lower blood pressure. Generic names of a few diuretics are Furosemide, Bumetanide, Metalazone, Hydrochlorothiazide, Spironolactone and Amiloride.

Some of the potential adverse effects of diuretics include hypotension, low levels of potassium in blood, rashes and muscle cramps.

Nitrates

Nitrates are medications given to treat angina. Nitrates dilate veins and arteries in the body including the coronary artery. Hence, they are also called vasodilators. This enables the heart to supply more blood through arteries that are partially blocked. Nitrates reduce arterial resistance against which the heart pumps blood into the arteries. This decreases its workload and oxygen demand. Nitrates are available in different forms – tablets that can be swallowed or placed under the tongue (sub-lingual), and buccal, where the pill has to be held between the cheek and gum or the lip and gum until it is dissolved. Nitroglycerin is also available as patches that can be stuck on the skin or topical ointments. A spray form is also available which is used at the beginning of an angina attack to reduce its duration and to prevent it from worsening. During a heart attack, nitroglycerin is administered intravenously. Generic names of a few nitrates are Nitroglycerin, Isosorbide dinitrate and Isosorbide mononitrate. Some of the adverse effects that nitrates can cause are headaches, dizziness, nausea and low blood pressure.

Inotropic Agents

Inotropic agents increase the energy with which the heart muscles contract. They are used to treat heart failure and some abnormal heart rhythms. Generic names of a few inotropic agents are Digoxin, Dopamine, Dobutamine and Digitoxin. Some of the side effects associated with digoxin are nausea, anorexia, vomiting, diarrhoea, headache, depression and visual disturbances. Dopamine and dobutamine may cause headaches, nausea and heart rhythm disturbances.

Lipid Lowering Agents

Since abnormal lipid levels contribute significantly to coronary artery disease, it is essential to keep them normal. Along with a healthy low-fat diet, these medications can be used to lower high cholesterol and triglyceride values. There are several classes of drugs that are used to treat hyperlipdemia such as HMG CoA reductase inhibitors, commonly known as statins and bile acid sequestrants. The common generic names of lipid lowering agents are Simvastatin, Fluvastatin, Atorvastatin, Nicotinic acid,

Cholestryramine, Gemfibrozil, Clofibrate and Fenofibrate. Some of the side effects associated with these drugs are abdominal pain or cramps, constipation, muscle weakness or pain and headache.

Invasive

Coronary artery disease takes decades to develop and produce symptoms. People may not always respond to medications and their symptoms may remain the same or worsen. In such cases, treatments to open up coronary arteries like angioplasty or bypass surgery are recommended. They might also be required when diagnostic tests show severe blockages and there is a higher risk of having a heart attack.

Revascularisation or restoring blood flow through the blocked coronary arteries to the heart muscles will reduce angina. Both angioplasty and bypass surgery has its own advantages and disadvantages. The doctor decides the suitable procedure based on patient's risk factors, medical conditions and complications.

An angioplasty or a bypass surgery is by no means a cure for coronary artery disease. Even after these procedures, medications and a healthy life style should be continued to prevent further development of this disease.

Coronary Angioplasty

Percutaneous Transluminal Coronary Angioplasty or PTCA is the complete medical term for angioplasty. This procedure, also known as Percutaneous Coronary Intervention or PCI, is usually performed by an interventional cardiologist in a cardiac catherisation laboratory. A catheter with a deflated balloon in the end, called the balloon catheter, is inserted into a blood vessel from the leg, arm or neck and passed all the way to the narrowed coronary artery. The balloon is then inflated to compress the plaque and open up the blocked artery.

A wire mesh tube called stent is placed in the artery to keep it open and reduce the probability of the artery narrowing again. Some stents are coated with medications to prevent narrowing. These are called drug-eluting stent. The others that are not coated are called bare-metal stents.

Patients may be advised to a bypass surgery instead of an angioplasty when they have multiple blockages, narrowing of arteries that are hard to reach by a catheter, left main coronary artery blockage and poor left ventricular function.

Heart attack patients need prompt treatment to open up blockages in the coronary arteries. The quicker their arteries are opened, the better their chances of survival are. Emergency coronary angioplasty is now a preferred way to remove blockages and prevent the heart muscles from dying. The time between the heart attack patient's arriving at the hospital to the time an angioplasty is done is called the 'Door to Balloon time'. The recommended door to balloon time by the American Heart Association is ninety minutes or less. Studies have shown that when the time to treatment is kept short, mortality rate is lower.

What to expect during an angioplasty?

For an elective angioplasty, you will be asked to fast for several hours before the procedure. You will be allowed to take medications ordered by your doctor with sips of water. You may be given an anti-platelet or anti-coagulant to decrease blood clotting around the catheter. A sedative may be given to ease your anxiety.

On the day of the procedure, an intravenous line will be placed. Electrode pads are placed on your chest and are connected to a machine to monitor your heart rate and rhythm. The area where the catheter is inserted is cleaned with antiseptic solution and local anaesthesia is injected at that site. General anaesthesia is not used for angioplasty and you will be awake during the procedure.

Once the incision area is numbed, the cardiologist will make a small cut and a short tube called sheath is inserted into the blood vessel. A catheter is threaded to the blocked artery and a small amount of contrast dye is injected. With the help of X-ray images, the exact location of the blockages is found. Then a balloon catheter is used to widen the blocked coronary artery. Chest pain may occur when the balloon is inflated but goes away when the balloon is deflated. The procedure may be repeated to treat multiple blockages. Most people having an angioplasty have stents placed in the site of the blockage. The stent will support the artery wall from collapsing or narrowing again. Depending on the number of blockages and any complications that may arise, an angioplasty can take half an hour to several hours.

Once the procedure is complete, you will be shifted to a recovery room. Your electrocardiogram will be monitored continuously. A nurse will check your vital signs and the catheter insertion site frequently. Once the sheath is removed, there will be pressure bandages and you must not bend your leg for several hours. Complete bed rest is required. This will prevent bleeding from the puncture site and help healing.

You may be discharged from the hospital in a day or two. Several medications including an anti-platelet will be prescribed. You may be asked to drink plenty of water to remove the dye from your body. There might be some restrictions with regards to exercise or carrying heavy objects. You must see a doctor at once if the puncture site is infected, painful or bleeding. You must also seek medical attention if you develop angina or shortness of breath.

Coronary angioplasty procedures have a high success rate. The overall risks associated with coronary angioplasty are very low. The chance of proceeding with emergency bypass surgery or having a heart attack is less than five per cent.

Bypass Surgery

Coronary Artery Bypass Graft (CABG) surgery, commonly known to nonmedical people as bypass surgery or heart bypass, is a major surgery and typically considered an open heart surgery performed by cardiothoracic surgeons. CABG is a procedure where veins or arteries elsewhere from the patient's body are used to create a detour for the blood to bypass the blockage in the coronary arteries. One end of the graft is usually sutured to the aorta and the other to the coronary artery beyond its blockage.

An artery from the chest called the internal mammary artery is commonly used to bypass the blockages in left anterior descending coronary artery. Saphenous vein from the leg or radial artery from the hand are also used as conduits for grafting other branches of the coronary artery.

During this procedure, the surgeon makes an incision in the middle of the chest. He then cuts the sternum open to get access to the heart and the aorta. He connects the heart to a heart-lung machine which takes over the function of oxygenating and pumping blood for a few minutes. The heart is stopped before grafting the veins and arteries to the coronary arteries. After the bypasses are complete, the heart is filled back with blood and it resumes its function. This method enables the surgeon to suture grafts in a still and bloodless setting with ease and safety.

An Off-Pump Coronary Artery Bypass surgery or OPCAB is a procedure where the heart-lung machine is not used. Instead the surgeon uses stabilising devices to hold the heart and performs the surgery on a beating heart. This method has gained popularity because all the side effects of using a heart lung machine are avoided and there is less recovery time. Sometimes, the surgeon can even work with a smaller-size incision, so that there is less scarring.

What to expect during a bypass surgery?

Most bypass surgeries are scheduled days or weeks ahead. You will be asked to get admitted in the hospital one day prior to the surgery. Your doctor will advise you to stop or change certain medications few days prior to the day of the surgery.

An angiogram done earlier will show the surgeons the exact locations of the blockages. An electrocardiogram, chest X-ray and routine blood tests are also performed, if not done recently. The surgeon and anaesthetist will meet you before surgery to explain the procedures and answer your questions. You will be on fasting after midnight and will be allowed to take your medications with sips of water. A pill to reduce anxiety is given. Chest, groin and legs will be shaved on the day of surgery. You may be asked to take a shower with a special soap to kill germs. An intravenous line will be started in your arm.

You will be awake when you enter the operation theatre and moved to the operating table. You may even remember the technicians putting on the oxygen mask. Medicines to put you under general anaesthesia will be given. An endotracheal tube is inserted into your windpipe through your nose or mouth. A ventilator will be connected when you are under general anaesthesia, a machine to help you breathe efficiently.

People who need multiple bypasses have veins taken from their legs or radial artery from their arms. After surgery you will have stitches on your chest, legs and/or arms. Two or more tubes called surgical drains are inserted. The tubes will help drain any blood or excess fluid that is collected in the chest cavity and prevent infection. These tubes will be removed within a day depending on the amount of fluid that is collected.

You may stay in the intensive care unit (ICU) for a day or two, provided there are no complications. There will be a lot of activity around you in the ICU with several machines beeping continuously. Your family will be allowed to visit you for a very short time. A team of doctors will keep visiting you and checking on your progress. You will be connected to several wires monitoring your electrocardiogram, heart rate, blood pressure and pressures in various heart chambers. Your intake and output of fluids will be closely monitored. You will be slowly weaned off the ventilators once the anaesthesia wears off. You start to breathe better on your own and cough and clear the secretions produced by the lungs. Once you are off the ventilator, oxygen will be supplemented through a face mask. The nurse will show you charts to communicate with you when you are connected to all the tubes. Your throat will be sore for a few days after the endotracheal tube is removed.

A physiotherapist will start working with you, encouraging you to cough and breathe deeper. You will be asked to keep a pillow on you chest while you cough. Chest physiotherapy also helps clear up lung secretions. You will be encouraged to get out of bed and start walking before you are sent to a normal ward. You may be enrolled in a cardiac rehabilitation program and a customised exercise plan will be given to you. A dietician works with you and suggests a diet suitable for you. Your appetite is usually very poor for several weeks after surgery. Decreased activity and less food can lead to constipation, too. There may be some swelling in the leg if vein was taken from there. Keeping the leg elevated and using compression stockings could reduce fluid accumulation.

Most sutures are absorbable and will dissolve on their own. Sometimes non-absorbable sutures or staples are used. They are normally removed in 5-7 days after surgery. If there are no complications, you will be discharged in a week to 10 days. At discharge time, you are given instructions on wound care and physical restrictions.

Chapter 7

Complications of a Heart Attack

Heart attack complications vary from person to person. Some may have a mild attack with no associated complications, while an extensive attack may lead to several complications. Complications may be prevented or minimised if the heart attack patients are treated immediately with an emergency angioplasty or thrombolytic therapy.

- **Heart Failure:** Part of the myocardium or the heart muscles die as a result of a heart attack. When the heart contracts these dead muscles do not pump along with the rest of the heart. This results in reduced blood pumping out of the heart. Heart failure results in fluid build up in the lungs, legs, ankles and feet. Congestion in the lungs can also occur.

- **Arrhythmias:** Arrhythmias are abnormal beatings of the heart. Since heart attacks cause scarring of the heart muscles, its electrical conduction system can be affected. Abnormal heart rhythms can also cause inefficient heart pumping. Cardiac arrest and ventricular fibrillation are abnormal rhythms that are fatal. Sometimes the sinus node or the pacemaker of the heart is affected and a pacemaker implantation becomes necessary.

- **Ventricular Aneurysm:** When a heart attack weakens the heart muscles, they dilate and bulge out to form an aneurysm. They often result in arrhythmias, inadequate cardiac output, heart failure and blood clots. People with aneurysms immediately after a heart attack have poor prognosis.

- **Clot Formation:** Clots can form in the heart chambers next to the affected heart muscles. They are more common when an aneurysm is present. Blood clots in the heart chambers can travel to the arteries of the brain or the heart, resulting in a stroke or another heart attack.

- **Ventricular Rupture:** This is one of the uncommon complications which often occur within a week after a heart attack. The heart attack may be so severe that the muscles rupture. The result of a rupture of a ventricular wall is catastrophic resulting in no blood circulation, shock and ultimately death.

Ventricular Septal Defect: When the wall between the two ventricles or the septum ruptures blood flows between the two ventricles. Ventricular septal defect occurs in about two per cent of people after a heart attack within 4-5 days. Chest pain returns and the general condition of the patient worsen. This defect is usually closed by surgery, but the clinical condition of the patient has to be stable.

Valve Regurgitation: Muscles attached to the heart muscles are called papillary muscles. When these structures are affected by the heart attack, it does not properly support the valves between the upper chambers and lower chambers of the heart. So blood leaks back into the atrium from the ventricles and reduce the amount of blood flowing out of the heart. Mitral valve regurgitation is also possible in patients who develop heart failure after a heart attack.

Recurrent Angina: When the artery that caused the heart attack gets blocked again causing reduced blood supply, chest pain occurs again. There may be blockages in other coronary arteries too. Angina after a heart attack may be temporary but continued ischemia will damage the heart muscles further. Reinfarction or another heart attack is also possible when the blockage completely closes off the blood supply to the myocardium.

- **Pericarditis:** The heart's outer layer is called a pericardium. Pericarditis is the inflammation of pericardium. People with pericarditis have sharp chest pain that changes with position and worsens with cough or breath. Other symptoms are fever, shortness of breath and dizziness. Aspirin or other non steroidal anti-inflammatory drugs are used to reduce the inflammation. Extra fluid accumulating around the heart may need removal by a procedure called pericardiectomy.

- **Cardiogenic Shock:** After a heart attack the blood flowing from the heart to the other organs may be poor. Organs like the brain, liver and kidneys suffer from inadequate oxygen supply. The body goes into a state of shock. Blood pressure in the body can be very low. This condition is an emergency. Medications are given to increase blood pressure and increase the heart's contractility. Some people may require a pacemaker implantation. A mechanical device called intra-aortic balloon pump is temporarily placed in the aorta may be used to improve the heart's function.

- **Depression:** Depression is very common after a heart attack. Depression hinders speedy recovery and increases the chances of death. Chronic undiagnosed and untreated depression affects everyday activities of patients. They experience more pain and fatigue. They are reluctant to eat properly or exercise well. Doctors should treat severe, chronic or recurrent depression. Medications may be required along with therapy in some patients.

Chapter 8

Prevention

A healthy natural heart is powerful than any medicine or treatment that science has given us. Since medications cannot guarantee a complete cure of coronary artery disease, preventing it is rational. To stop before it begins and control once it begins is the best approach to combat coronary heart disease. You can achieve effective prevention if you start making lifestyle changes early.

Several decades ago heart attacks were associated with old age alone. But now several risk factors have been identified that cause heart attacks and decrease lifespan. If lifestyle changes are made to minimise these risk factors, heart disease can be prevented. Prevention is not only better than cure, but it is also cheaper. Medications and diagnostics tests are much more expensive than eating healthy or joining a gym. It is also important to educate young adults about the negative effects of tobacco and drugs. They should learn to reject them and build a healthy world.

Prevention can be classified as primary and secondary prevention. Primary prevention is the effort to modify the risk factors so that the development of coronary heart disease is delayed. Secondary prevention aims at preventing a heart attack or death in patients with coronary heart disease. In secondary prevention, medications are given to both treat heart disease and control risk factors.

There should be no compromise when it comes to health and preventing or reversing coronary heart disease lies mostly in your hands. With the help of your doctor assess your risk factors and talk about preventive measures. Some of the risk factors increase your risk way higher than others. The more your risk factors, the higher your chances of heart attacks. So it becomes necessary to prevent or control immediately. You may not be able to change all your habits at once. Make one change at a time and constantly remind yourself to keep up the good. Healthy living makes you energetic and younger. You become motivated and happy.

Stop Smoking

Your doctors will explain the risk factors associated with smoking and encourage you to quit it. When you are ready to quit smoking fix a quit date which is realistic. You should be able to wean down and stop smoking completely by that date. Create new goals in life that will require you to stay healthy and keep you away from cigarettes. Identify the things that motivate you, for example your kids or family. Focus on them and remind yourself that they require you to be fit and healthy.

The problem most people face with quitting is not quitting itself but not smoking again. If you restart smoking, don't think of it as a failure. Don't fret or fear relapse as they give you a chance for you to rectify and prevent future relapses.

Initially remove things that you associate with smoking like ashtrays at home or your favourite cigarette lighter. Whenever possible, stay away from people who smoke. Even second-hand smokes can create an urge for you to reach a cigarette. Tell your family and friends that you intent to quit smoking and you need their support. Believe you can quit.

Some of you may require nicotine patch or gum or medications such as bupropion to stop smoking. Other things that can aid you to control your need of a cigarette are support groups, hypnotherapy and acupuncture.

Heart-Healthy Diet

Healthy eating habits can prevent numerous diseases. Eating habits start early. So it is important to feed a child healthy and teach young adults to follow a healthy diet. You must also eat just enough calories to maintain a healthy weight. Too much food, even healthy food, can make you gain weight. Foods that are known to increase the risk factors for heart diseases should be used sparingly.

Foods high in cholesterol and saturated fat should be avoided or limited. Less than 30 per cent of the total calories should be from fat. Cholesterol intake should be not more than 300 milligrams a day. Monosaturated and polysaturated fats may help lower your total body cholesterol; but it must be used in moderation.

Proteins should be added to each meal. Choose proteins from low-fat sources such as lean meat, skinless chicken legs, fish, soy products and legumes. Full fat milk, sausages and bacon are examples of proteins to avoid or limit.

Fruits and vegetables should be a huge part of your diet. You must have atleast 5 – 6 servings of fruits and vegetables a day. They are low in calories, rich in fibre and vitamins. Bright coloured fruits and vegetables such as carrots and blue berries are rich in antioxidants that fight heart disease and cancer.

Whole grains are a good source of carbohydrates compared to refined forms. They provide more fibre and are absorbed more slowly in blood than simple sugars. For example whole wheat flour is better than refined flour and brown rice is better than white rice. Avoid cakes and other pastries which are made from refined flour and are high in sugar and fat.

Plan and create menus ahead. This will help you to think of what you are eating and making sure that it is a complete balanced diet. You can make sure that you are getting all the nutrients you need from your food. A variety of foods can be included in your meals and snacks if you plan for the week.

Do not forget to drink eight to ten glasses of water everyday. When you wait till you are thirsty to drink a glass of water, that means your body is already dehydrated. Every cell function requires water and is essential for all vital functions. Water removes toxins from the body. Hydration boosts your immune system and your energy levels. It can help speed up recovery process in both internal and external injury. Drnking sufficient water helps reduce hypertension, lose weight, treat depression and sleep disorders. It improves better blood supply to your skin, so it remains healthy and good looking. Water is also known to prevent some forms of cancer.

Control Hypertension

Hypertension is not only known to cause coronary heart disease, but also strokes, kidney disease, peripheral artery disease and retinopathy. It is very important to keep you blood pressure as close to the normal range as possible. The systolic blood pressure or the top number should be less than 120 mmHg and the diastolic blood pressure should be less than 80 mmHg. If your blood pressure is normal, check it atleast once or twice a year. If you have hypertension, you should check your blood pressure atleast once a month to make sure it is under control.

Many who are recently diagnosed with hypertension are able to lower their blood pressure readings without medications by making some simple changes in their life.

Salt or sodium affects your blood pressure. Excess salt is hidden in many processed foods. Recognise foods that are known to contain high amount of sodium and limit it. Eat less than 2 gm of sodium per day.

Other things that can help lower blood pressure are

- Weight reduction
- Regular Exercise

- Limiting your alcohol intake
- Diet rich in potassium and sodium
- Managing stress

If these lifestyle changes fail to maintain your blood pressure, you may need medications to lower it. There are a number of medications to treat hypertension. Your physician may start a medication and continue to monitor your blood pressure for a few months. They may suggest you buy a home monitor and keep a record of your daily blood pressure. Depending on the values he may increase or decrease the dosage. They may even replace or add another medication to get better control.

Once you've reached normal values, you should continue to monitor your blood pressure and ensure it is controlled well. You may need to take your medications for a very long time. Do not stop taking your pills without your doctor's advice.

Control Cholesterol

Abnormal cholesterol and triglyceride levels are one of the most important risk factors for heart attacks. Many patients with abnormal lipid levels often respond to a low fat diet. Make changes that you can keep up and avoid drastic changes. Use low fat milk instead of whole milk. Avoid foods high in saturated fats. Add more fibre to your diet.

Eat foods that can provide antioxidants such as fruits and vegetables with vitamin C, vitamin E and beta carotene. Take omega-3 and omega-6 fats which can help lower bad cholesterol. A clove of garlic a day may lower cholesterol level. Losing weight and regular aerobic exercise can also lower cholesterol levels. Niacin, also called Vitamin B3, can lower the bad cholesterol and increase the good cholesterol.

When cholesterol and triglyceride values are high because of a genetic problem, diet and exercise may not be sufficient to keep them normal. Your doctor will prescribe medications depending on your lab values. There are several groups of medications that can lower lipids. Talk to your doctor about the side effects of these medications. Statins, commonly used to treat dyslipidemia, may cause some liver or kidney damage. So you may be required to have periodical blood tests to check your liver function and kidney function.

Desirable Lipid Levels

Total cholesterol – Less than 200 mg/dl

LDL cholesterol – Less than 130 mg/dl

[People with risk for heart disease should lower their LDL values to less than 100 mg/dl]

HDL cholesterol – Above 40 mg/dl

[Higher than 60 mg/dl is better]

Triglycerides – Less than 150 mg/dl

Control Diabetes

Since diabetics are three times more likely to suffer from coronary artery disease, it is important to maintain your sugar levels near normal at all times possible. Carbohydrate is an important part of our diet, but it causes a rise in blood sugar levels. Learn about serving sizes and limit the amount of carbohydrates to a maximum of 11 servings per day. Add proteins to every meal and reduce fat intake. Eat small meals at regular intervals. Exercise and weight loss have also proven to lower blood sugar levels.

Check your blood sugar levels at home. Fasting blood sugar should be under 100mg for non-diabetic people and less than 130 mg/dl for diabetics. Blood sugar level after 2 hours of a meal should be less than 140 mg/dl for non-diabetics and less than 180mg/dl for diabetics. Haemoglobin A1C should be tested atleast once in three months. Normal HbA1C is under 6 per cent and less than 7 per cent means good control of diabetes.

Medications to lower blood sugar levels may be necessary in people with Type II diabetes when lifestyle changes are not enough. Type I diabetics will need insulin injection everyday to regulate their blood sugar levels. Visit your doctor regularly to make sure you are under good control. Since diabetics are prone to foot ulcers, have a foot examination during your physical. Get an eye examination every year and a dental check twice a year.

Maintain Healthy Weight

Your body weight increases your chances of having several illnesses such as diabetes, hypertension, high cholesterol, joint disorders, heart disease and stroke. So it is very important to maintain a healthy weight. Along with keeping your Body Mass Index (BMI) normal, you must also reduce abdominal obesity. A large waist increases the risk of mortality.

Regular exercise and a low fat diet can help achieve weight loss. If you are having trouble losing weight, talk to a dietician. Maintain a food diary to track what you ate and see what you can do to eat better.

Weight loss needs a lot of commitment and once you reach your desired weight, you must continue to maintain it. Fad diets may help you lose weight faster but the results may not last. If you lose weight very fast, there are chances that you will gain them back on. Only a proper balanced diet along with moderate physical exercise can provide steady weight loss.

Regular Exercise

The benefits of exercise are enormous. It strengthens the heart and lungs. Along with burning body fat, it can strengthen muscles. Proper aerobic and strengthening exercise makes your bones stronger. There is increased oxygen supply to every organ in your body including the skin. More oxygen supply to the brain enhances memory and thinking. More toxins are removed from the body. Stress hormones are lowered, so the blood vessels are relaxed and blood pressure is lowered. Endorphins, known as happy hormones, are increased with exercise.

Adults should do moderate physical exercise for a minimum of thirty minutes at least three times a week. A brisk walking, light jogging, swimming, gardening, bicycle riding and certain sports such as softball and volley ball are considered as moderate intensity exercises. In addition to this resistance exercises about twice a week can increase muscle endurance. Weight training and climbing steps are examples of resistance exercise.

Reduce Stress

Stress raises your heart rate and blood pressure. The hormones released during stress can affect the heart and arteries. Reducing or avoiding stress is probably the most difficult problem we face today. You should learn to deal and balance problems in different situations. Identify the true causes of your stress and closely observe your attitude and habits trying to deal with it. You may be able to just completely avoid certain causes. Some are temporary and is probably because you are trying to too many things at the same time.

Drinking, smoking, overeating, isolation, sleeping a lot, angry outbursts and medicines to relax may reduce stress temporarily but causes more harm later. Healthier ways to manage stress are by avoiding the stress when possible. For example, accepting more work than you can handle can add more stress to your life. So, learn to say no when you've reached your limits. Share household responsibilities among your family members. Try to change the situation if possible and learn to compromise when necessary. If stressful situations cannot be changed, try a different and positive perspective. Do not react to all uncontrollable problems. Talk about your problem to your family, friends or a therapist. They can probably help you get through the challenge.

Try relaxation techniques such as a long walk, listening to music, working out or a massage. Aromatherapy can help some to relax. Find time to do things that you enjoy the most, such as playing an instrument, painting, gardening or dancing.

Avoid caffeine, high sugar foods, alcohol, cigarettes and drugs. They worsen stress in long run. Adequate sleep is very important in coping with stress. A good night sleep will replenish your body and help you perform better the next day.

Chapter 9
Cardio Pulmonary Resuscitation (CPR)

Heart muscle or myocardium suffers severe oxygen starvation during a heart attack and often results in scarring of tissues. These scar tissues impair the normal electrical conduction of the heart causing abnormal heart rhythm or arrhythmia. Severe arrhythmia impairs effective contraction of the heart and reduces blood flow to the vital organs.

A condition called **sudden cardiac arrest** is when the heart stops beating unexpectedly. A cardiac arrest is most likely to occur in patients with coronary artery disease or with certain types of arrhythmia. A person who suffers a cardiac arrest will lose consciousness and have no pulse or breathing. Sudden cardiac death can occur with minutes unless his heart is forced back to pumping in a normal rhythm. The chances of survival are better if an **automated external defibrillator (AED)** is used within five minutes of collapse. An AED delivers an appropriate amount of shock to the heart to restart it. However an AED may not be available at all situations. CPR or even chest compressions is the next best option to improve survival rate and buy time until emergency help arrives.

Cardiopulmonary resuscitation (CPR) is a life saving emergency procedure that involves compressing the heart manually through the chest wall and breathing into their nose or mouth. Chest compressions cause a small amount of blood to flow to the vital organs. The chest needs to be compressed about 2 inches deep with both hands at the rate of 100 compressions per minute. *An effective CPR provided immediately can double the chances of survival.* Remember to push hard and fast. Slow, interrupted or shallow compressions may not improve the chances of survival.

How to do CPR

The guidelines for adult cardiopulmonary resuscitation are in this order – C A B.

C stands for Circulation

A stands for Airway

B stands for Breathing

When a person becomes unconscious, ask someone to call for an ambulance immediately or do it yourself if you are alone. Check the person to see if he is breathing and his heart is still pumping. Pulse can be found in the carotid artery which is located in the neck by placing your fingers on either sides of the windpipe. In case of an absent pulse, start chest compressions immediately.

Circulation

- Chest compressions can restore blood circulation to the the brain and other vital organs.
- Place the victim on his back on a firm flat surface and kneel beside him.
- Keeping your elbows straight place the heel of your one hand over the person's chest between his nipples. Keep the second hand on top of the first.
- Push the chest down about 2 inches keeping your hands straight and using your upper body weight.
- Compressions should be about 100 per minute or time yourself to two compressions per second.

- Continue with the chest compressions until the emergency medical personnel arrive or the patient becomes conscious.

Airway

When atleast 30 chest compressions are performed, you can proceed to clearing the airway.

- Placing your palm on the victims's forehead tilt his head back and lift his chin forward with the other hand. It is called the head-tilt, chin-lift maneuver. This opens his airway.

- Place your cheek and ear close to face and feel for his breath listening to breath sounds, check his chest for motion with breath. When you find no breath or he isn't breathing normally administer mouth to mouth respiration.

Breathing

Rescue breathing is normally given through mouth to mouth. When a person has serious mouth injury or if his mouth cannot be opened mouth to nose breath can be given as well.

- After tilted the head and the chin pushed forward, pinch the victim's nostril and cover his mouth with yours making a seal.

- Give two rescue breaths. Each breath should last for about a second.
- Go back to chest compressions as soon as two breaths are given.

When there are more than one of you to help, one person can do compressions while the other performs the breathing. Two breaths are given after every thirty chest compressions. However, if you untrained or are unsure of giving mouth to mouth breaths continue chest compressions alone. Even untrained responders are recommended to perform chest compressions. It is called **hands-only CPR**. When the victim groans or becomes conscious you can stop performing CPR and place him in recovery position. Lay him on his side allowing him to keep his airway open and preventing him to choke on his own saliva.

CPR saves lives. Educate yourself to perform CPR because you may find yourself in a situation of need and not know what to do. Even children can learn and perform effective CPR. Voluntary humanitarian organisations provide CPR training classes for everyone.

Glossary

- ACE-inhibitors - Angiotensin Converting Enzyme (ACE) inhibitors are mainly used to treat hypertension.
- Anaphylaxis - It is a life threatening allergic reaction.
- Aneurysm - Aneurysm is a dilated artery wall.
- Angina – Chest pain caused due to coronary artery disease
- Angiogram – An invasive test that uses X-ray to diagnose diseases in the blood vessels.
- Angioplasty – A catheterisation procedure that is used to widen narrowed blood vessels.
- Antioxidants – Substances that can reduce cell damage caused by free radicals.
- Anti-platelets – Anti-platelets are medications used to decrease platelet aggregation and prevent clot formation.
- Aorta – Aorta, the largest artery in the body, originates from the left ventricle.
- Arrhythmias – Arrhythmias are abnormal rate or rhythms of the heartbeats.
- Atherosclerosis – Atherosclerosis is fatty deposits in the artery walls that block blood flow.

- Atrium – Atrium is the upper chamber of the heart. Plural of atrium is atria.
- Autoimmune – Autoimmune refers to the body's immune system acting against its own cells and tissues.
- Beta blockers – Beta blockers or beta adrenergic blockers are used to treat hypertension, arrhythmias and chest pain.
- Calcium channel blockers – Calcium channel blockers are drugs used to treat hypertension and angina.
- Cardiac arrest – Cardiac arrest means the heart stops beating suddenly causing no blood circulation and when untreated sudden death within minutes.
- Cardiac output – Cardiac output is the amount of blood that is pumped by the ventricles in a minute.
- Cardiogenic shock – Cardiogenic shock is a state of emergency where the heart does not pump enough blood to meet the demands of the body.
- Cardiomyopathy – Cardiomyopathy is the disease of the heart muscle.
- Catheterization – Catheterization means inserting a catheter into your blood vessel or body cavity.
- Coronary artery – The artery that supplies the heart.
- CRP – C-reactive protein (CRP) is protein produced by the liver whose levels in blood increases with inflammation.
- Diuretics – Diuretics are medicines used to treat hypertension and heart failure by excreting more water and sodium from the body.
- Dyslipidemia – Dyslipidemia is abnormal levels of lipids in the blood.

- Dyspnoea – Dyspnoea means difficulty in breathing.
- Emboli – Emboli are blood clots that travel from the heart or one blood vessel to another blood vessel. The singular form of emboli is embolus.
- Endocarditis – Endocarditis is inflammation of the inner layer of the heart and valves.
- *Endocardium – Endocardium is the inner layer of the heart.*
- Epicardium – Epicardium is the outer layer of the heart.
- Fibrinogen – Fibrinogen is a protein that helps in blood coagulation process.
- HDL – High density lipoprotein (HDL) also known as good cholesterol helps clear blockages in the arteries.
- Heart failure – Heart failure is the inability of the heart to pump enough blood to the body.
- Homocysteine – Homocystiene is an amino acid that is synthesised in the body.
- Hyperglycaemia – Hyperglycaemia is the increased levels of sugar in blood.
- Hypertension – Hypertension means high blood pressure.
- Hyperthyroidism – Hyperthyroidism is overproduction of thyroid hormone.
- Hypoglycaemia – Hypoglycaemia means low levels of sugar in blood.
- Hypotension – Hypotension means low blood pressure.
- Hypothyroidism – Hypothyroidism means underproduction of thyroid horome.
- Infarction – Infarction means localised necrosis or death of cells caused by reduced blood supply.

- Invasive – Invasive means procedure that involves skin puncture or inserting an instrument into the body.
- Ischaemia – Ischaemia means insufficient blood supply to any muscle or organ.
- LDL – LDL or low density lipoprotein also known as bad cholesterol is known to cause blockages in arteries.
- Lumen – Lumen means the cavity of a blood vessel.
- Mediastinum – Mediastinum is the compartment of the thorax that contains several structures including the heart, aorta and pulmonary artery.
- Mitral valve – Mitral valve is the valve between the left atrium and left ventricle.
- Myocardial infarction – Myocardial Infarction means heart attack.
- Myocardium – Myocardium means heart muscle.
- Nitrates – Nitrates are medicines used to treat chest pain.
- Pericarditis – Pericarditis means inflammation of the pericardium.
- Pericardium – Pericardium is a thin sac that encloses the heart.
- Peripheral artery disease – Peripheral artery disease is the narrowing of peripheral blood vessels.
- Pulmonary artery – Pulmonary artery carries deoxygenated blood from the heart to the lungs.
- Pulmonary valve – Pulmonary valve is the valve between the right ventricle and the pulmonary artery.
- Renal insufficiency – Renal insufficiency or renal failure is the inability of the kidneys to function properly.

- Retinopathy – Retinopathy means disease of the retina of the eye.
- Sepsis – Sepsis is a potentially serious medical condition caused by infection entering the blood stream.
- Septum – Septum is the wall separating the heart into left and right sides.
- Thrombolysis – Thrombolysis means breaking and dissolving blood clots.
- Thrombolytic agents – Thrombolytic agents are drugs that are used to break clots in the blood vessels.
- Thrombus – Thrombus is a blood clot in the blood vessels or in the heart.
- Tricupsid valve – Tricuspid valve is the valve between the right atrium and right ventricle.
- Valve regurgitation – Valve regurgitation or insufficiency is a condition where the valve allows back flow of blood from one chamber into another.
- Ventricle – Ventricle is the lower chamber of the heart.

References

1. Coronary Vasospasm as a Possible Cause of Myocardial Infarction — A Conclusion Derived from the Study of Preinfarction Angina. Attilio Maseri, M.D., Antonio L'Abbate, M.D., et al. N Engl J Med 1978; 299:1271-1277
2. Plaque fissuring- the cause of acute myocardial infarction, sudden ischaemic death, and crescendo angina. Michael J Davies, Anthony C Thomas. Br Heart J 1985;53:362-373
3. Causes of Myocardial Infarction. Domingo Baitlon. JAMA. 1975;233(13):1357
4. Effect of Beta-Blockade on Mortality among High-Risk and Low-Risk Patients after Myocardial Infarction. Stephen S. Gottlieb, M.D., Robert J. McCarter, Sc.D., and Robert A. Vogel, M.D. N Engl J Med 1998; 339:489-497
5. Hemostatic Factors and the Risk of Myocardial Infarction or Sudden Death in Patients with Angina Pectoris. Simon G. Thompson, M.A., Joachim Kienast, M.D., et al. N Engl J Med 1995; 332:635-64
6. Primary Angioplasty for Acute Myocardial Infarction — Is It Worth the Wait?
7. Alice K. Jacobs, M.D. N Engl J Med 2003; 349:798-800August 21, 2003
8. Klein I, Ojamaa K. Thyroid hormone and the cardiovascular system. N Engl J Med 2001 Feb 15;344(7):501-9.

9. Thrombolysis, Peripheral: Evan J Samett, Ali Nawaz Khan. Lancet. 2003 Jan 4;361(9351):13-20.
10. Primary angioplasty versus intravenous thrombolytic therapy for acute myocardial infarction: a quantitative review of 23 randomised trials. Keeley EC, Boura JA, Grines CL. Circulation. 2010;121:1484-1491.
11. Cardiac complications of mediastinal radiotherapy. Benjamin F. Byrd, III, MD, FACC and Lisa A. Mendes, MD, FACC. J Am Coll Cardiol, 2003; 42:750-751
12. Screening for Coronary Artery Disease After Mediastinal Irradiation for Hodgkin's Disease. Paul A. Heidenreich, Ingela Schnittger, etal. Journal of Clinical Oncology, Vol 25, No 1 (January 1), 2007: pp. 43-49
13. Primary Angioplasty Versus Fibrinolysis in Acute Myocardial Infarction
14. Long-Term Follow-Up in the Danish Acute Myocardial Infarction 2 Trial
15. Peter H. Nielsen; Michael Maeng, MD, PhD, et al. Circulation. 2010;121:1484-1491
16. Peter Damman, Marcel A.M. Beijk, Wichert J. Kuijt, etal.
17. Multiple Biomarkers at Admission Significantly Improve the Prediction of Mortality in Patients Undergoing Primary Percutaneous Coronary Intervention for Acute ST-Segment Elevation Myocardial Infarction
18. J Am Coll Cardiol 2011 57: 29-36.
19. Gibbons RJ, Abrams J, Chatterjee K, et al. ACC/AHA 2002 guideline update for the management of patients with chronic stable angina - summary article: a report of the American college of Cardiology/ American Heart Association Task Force on practice guidelines (Committee on the Management of Patients with Chronic Stable Angina). J Am Coll Cardilol 2003;41(1) 159-168.

20. Henry Shih, Brian Lee, Randall J. Lee, and Andrew J. Boyle
21. The Aging Heart and Post-Infarction Left Ventricular Remodeling
22. J Am Coll Cardiol 2011 57: 9-17.
23. Saif S Rathore, Jeptha P Curtis,et al. Association of door-to-balloon time and mortality in patients admitted to hospital with ST elevation myocardial infarction: national cohort study. BMJ 2009; 338:b1807
24. "Toothbrushing, inflammation, and risk of cardiovascular disease: results from Scottish Health Survey" BMJ, 27 May 2010
25. American Heart Association. Evidence-Based Guidelines for Cardiovascular Disease Prevention in Women: 2007 Update. Circulation. 2007;115:1481-1501
26. Primary cardiac sarcoma: reports of two cases and a review of current literature
27. Mohan P Devbhandari, Shaista Meraj, Mark T Jones, Isaac Kadir and Ben Bridgewater
28. Journal of Cardiothoracic Surgery 2007, 2:34 doi:10.1186/1749-8090-2-34
29. Primary Prevention of Coronary Heart Disease: Guidance From Framingham
30. A Statement for Healthcare Professionals From the AHA Task Force on Risk Reduction
31. Scott M. Grundy, MD, PhD, Chair; Gary J. Balady, MD, et al. Circulation. 1998;97:1876-1887
32. Kidney Disease and Heart Attacks
33. http://www.annals.org/content/137/7/I-12.full

Books

1. Braunwald's Heart Disease: A Textbook of Cardiovascular Medicine.

2. The ultimate guide to heart health: Mayo Clinic.
3. American Heart Association's Guide to Heart Attack - Treatment, Recovery and Prevention.
4. Prevention Of Myocardial Infarction by Joann E. Manson, Paul M. Ridker, J. Michael Gazino, Charles H. Hennekens.
5. Catecholamines and heart disease By Pallab K. Ganguly.

Websites

www.webmd.com/
www. theheart.org/
www.clevelandclinic.org/heartcenter
www.nhlbi.nih.gov
www.americanheart.org
www.womenheart.org
httpp://heart.healthcentersonline.com
http://www.hc-sc.gc.ca/hl-vs/iyh-vsv/life-vie/dent-eng.php
http://www.webmd.com/heart-disease/features/hope-for-heart-advances-in-treatment
http://www.ftc.gov/os/comments/cigarettetesting/536798-00019.pdf
http://www.cdc.gov/tobacco/basic_information/health_effects/heart_disease/index.htm
http://emedicine.medscape.com/article/162449-overview
http://atvb.ahajournals.org/cgi/content/full/atvbaha;20/9/2167
http://www.drkaslow.com/html/fibrinogen.html
http://www.nytimes.com/2006/03/14/health/14real.html